"In *A Surgeon's Book of Hope* I decided to write about some of the patients I'd treated, or had been treated by doctors I knew, and who had survived despite the long odds against them. Maybe, I thought, reading about patients who had beaten the odds, survived and thrived when we wise physicians 'knew' they couldn't, might give someone who needed it a lift. I know that just reviewing these cases and reliving them mentally has been a stimulating, happy experience for me. I hope it will prove to be as pleasant for the reader."

—WILLIAM A. NOLEN, M.D.

"THE HUMAN SIDE OF MEDICINE . . . ENCOURAGEMENT FOR ALL READERS."

—*JACKSON TENNESSEE SUN*

A Surgeon's Book of Hope

William A. Nolen, M.D.

BERKLEY BOOKS, NEW YORK

This Berkley book contains the complete
text of the original hardcover edition.
It has been completely reset in a type face
designed for easy reading, and was printed
from new film.

A SURGEON'S
BOOK OF HOPE

A Berkley Book / published by arrangement with
Coward, McCann & Geoghegan, Inc.

PRINTING HISTORY
Coward, McCann & Geoghegan edition / July 1980
Berkley edition / June 1982

ISBN: 0-425-05334-2

A BERKLEY BOOK® TM 757,375
Berkley Books are published by Berkley Publishing Corporation,
200 Madison Avenue, New York, New York 10016.
The name "BERKLEY" and the stylized "B" with design
are trademarks belonging to Berkley Publishing Corporation.
PRINTED IN THE UNITED STATES OF AMERICA

*To the memory of Mary Davidson, R.N.,
who showed all of us who knew her
what courage really is.*

Contents

This is a work of nonfiction, one man's view of the world suggested by his experiences.

Introduction

The work of a practicing physician is always challenging, frequently gratifying, often joyful. There are, however, occasions when it becomes very depressing. As one of my partners, Dr. Harold Wilmot, said to me shortly after I had moved to Litchfield, Minnesota, "Bill, this is a darn tough business. The worst of it is that you know, even though you may win a lot of battles, eventually you're going to lose the war. Everybody dies."

He's right, of course, but that hasn't stopped Harold, who celebrated his eightieth birthday in 1978 and still carries on a busy general practice, from continuing the fight. He has helped a lot of patients win a lot of battles, and that's really what the practice of medicine is all about.

In January 1979, I talked to Lennox Danielson one morning as we stood in the small kitchen near the operating room, having a cup of coffee after finishing an operation on eighty-seven-year-old Hilda Jackson. We'd found that she had a cancer of the pancreas the size of a small grapefruit. It was stuck to some major blood vessels that couldn't be sacrificed so I had had to leave the tumor behind, but I had been able to sew her intestine to her stomach and gall bladder so that whatever time she had left to live she'd be able to live in comfort. "Lennox," I asked, "how long have you been in practice?"

"Almost forty-seven years," he said. "I went into practice with my dad in 1932." Lennox is seventy-five and has lived in Litchfield all his life. He's a rugged man with a busy general practice. He's certainly one of the best hunters in Litchfield and, even at seventy-five, he'd no more think of buying a cord of split wood than he would a new Cadillac; he still splits the logs himself. Six years ago he bought a slightly used Oldsmobile, which we all call affectionately the "gray ghost." He has put 125,000 miles on it, a lot of it on drives to the farms outside of town. He's one of the few of us who make house calls without griping.

"Doesn't this business ever get you down?" I asked. "Wasn't it more fun practicing back in the early thirties?"

He looked at me as though I'd asked two silly questions. "Sure, it sometimes gets me down," he said, "I've lived long enough to see a lot of my old patients—patients who were my friends—die. But that's the way life is. You do the best you can and sometimes you help people.

"And as far as medical practice being more fun in the old days than it is now, that's a lot of nonsense. Heck, in the old days you'd spend half a day getting out to some farm to deliver a baby and if anything went wrong—say the mother hemorrhaged—you'd be lucky if you could get her back to the hospital before she died. Even if you made it you probably wouldn't be able to save her; blood transfusions were mighty rare in those days.

"And the patients you'd see with pneumonia—what could you do for them? Nothing, really. I'd feed them aspirin and maybe tell them to use a mustard plaster, but they either made it through the crisis or they didn't. Now we give them penicillin or some other antibiotic and they're well before you know it. No thanks. I wouldn't want to go back to the 'good old days' for anything. I like being able to help people."

Lennox cheered me up temporarily, but then I thought again of Mrs. Jackson; her chances of being cured, even with the new anticancer drugs, were just about zero. I asked Lennox if that didn't bother him.

"Sure, it does," he said, "but she's had eighty-seven pretty good years and we'll see to it, until she dies, that she isn't uncomfortable.

"And you know, Bill, there's one thing about medicine you shouldn't forget; nothing is certain. How long have you been here? Nineteen years, isn't it?"

"Right," I said. I'd arrived in Litchfield to begin practice as the only general surgeon in Meeker County on the first of August in 1960.

"Well then, you've seen patients whom you've given up on bounce back, haven't you? Heck, I know you have; I've worked with you on some of them. Remember Joanna Roberts, the one who had ovarian cancer? We didn't think she'd last six months. That was one of the first cases you did for me, so it has to be almost nineteen years since we operated. I saw her in my office just last week when she brought one of her grandchildren in with a cold. Every time I've seen her over these last nineteen years, I remember how we told her husband Al that her case was hopeless and how dismal he and her kids were. Well, she fooled us, didn't she? She and I always have a chuckle over how wrong you and I were.

"Bill, you know as well as I do that Hilda Jackson will probably die of that pancreatic tumor. We helped her as much as we could, but there are limits to what we can do. But you also know we could be wrong. She might last another ten years. She might beat that cancer. I'll admit her chances of making it aren't good, but they aren't zero either. Think back over your work here. Think of some of the patients you figured couldn't possibly survive. I'll bet you'll be able to recollect dozens who have fooled you. I know I can think of plenty who surprised me."

Later that day I began, mentally, to review some of the cases that I'd seen over the last nineteen years. Heaven knows, there had been a lot of them. As the only board certified surgeon in the county I'd done an awful lot of operating, probably close to 6000 cases, if I included the hernias, hemorrhoids and appendectomies.

And, since for most of those years there have been only about a dozen doctors on the active hospital staff—all, except me, in family practice—we'd been a pretty close-knit group. I work most often with my six partners in the Litchfield Clinic, but I've done the major surgery for the four other private practitioners. In our ninety-two bed rural hospital—the Meeker County Hospital—anytime anyone on the staff has an "interesting" case all the other doctors hear about it. As I thought back over the years, I certainly could think of a lot of patients who, by all the standard medical criteria, shouldn't have survived but did.

Additionally, as I reviewed not only my years of practice but my years of surgical training at Bellevue, I could think of a lot of advances that had been made in medicine. When I graduated from Tufts Medical School in 1953 and went off to Bellevue for five years of surgical training (interrupted from 1955 to 1957 by two years of service in the Army Medical Corps), tuberculosis was still widespread; it was almost routine for one intern or resident to contract the disease each year. Polio cases were a dime a dozen. Measles encephalitis occasionally reared its ugly head. Now, in 1980, these diseases were virtually nonexistent. The thoracic surgeons, who had spent most of their time operating on patients with tuberculosis, were now busy doing open heart surgery with mortality rates of only a fraction of one percent.

In other fields we'd come an equally long way. When I was at Bellevue we used to say of leukemia patients "either six weeks, six months or six years"—that was the average life span depending on whether the patient had an acute, subacute or chronic form of the disease. In 1980 most patients were not only surviving for many years but some—using the standard criterion of five-year survival without any treatment and no evidence of recurring disease—had been cured.

The orthopedic surgeons, who before the antibiotic era had spent much of their time removing pieces of dead bone from patients with chronic osteomyelitis (bone infection), were now busily replacing arthritic hips and knees with new joints made of metals and alloys that hadn't even been *discovered* twenty years ago.

And in the last five years we have seen dramatic gains in the ability of doctors to successfully reattach severed limbs. Ten years ago we could occasionally restore an arm cut off above the elbow or a leg separated in the area of the mid-thigh. At these levels the blood vessels and nerves are large enough so that the surgeon can see them with his naked eye or ordinary glasses. But farther down the limb the caliber of these structures is so small that it was usually impossible to satisfactorily join the ends together. Reattachment might be attempted, but it was usually necessary to amputate the foot or hand a few days later because of the onset of gangrene.

Then, in about 1975, surgeons began using microscopes in their work. These microscopes, which are generally used with a magnification of 16X to 25X, enabled them smoothly to reunite the tiny nerves and blood vessels that couldn't be seen without magnification. In 1977, for example, a testicle was transplanted from one identical twin to his brother, who had been born without either testicle. Surgery on the small vessels that supply the testicle (the artery measured only 0.5 millimeters in diameter) would have been impossible without the very fine synthetic suture materials developed in the last few years.

Fingers and toes have been reattached after amputation. At the 1979 meeting of the American College of Surgeons, one of the few minor arguments was between those surgeons who felt that, in an adult, reattachment of a single toe or finger was probably unnecessary. It is simpler to close the amputated site than to spend the two or three hours of reattachment of bone, tendon, nerves and arteries takes, and most patients would probably prefer the almost immediate use of the hand that amputation allowed to going through the prolonged convalescence that replantation requires. Assuming the finger or toe was suitable for reattachment, i.e., not crushed at the end so the vessels were unusable, it was generally agreed that the decision should be left to the patient (as, of course, it always is). Agreement was unanimous that, in children, strong recommendations for reattachment should be made.

And as for the obstetricians, the premature two- and three-pound babies who inevitably died twenty years ago are now frequently saved. We even have a new group of specialists, the perinatologists, pediatricians with special training in the care of high-risk newborn premature infants. The perinatologists are just one more of the vast number of subspecialists that have come into existence in the last twenty years, simply because the explosion of medical knowledge has been so great that it has become increasingly difficult to master more than a small part of it. The family practitioners, however, are new specialists, who manage to take care of most routine ailments very competently and, equally important, to identify the patients who need the help of a subspecialist.

Who knows, I thought that January afternoon, maybe tomorrow or next week or next month someone will announce the discovery of a drug that will melt away Mrs. Jackson's pancreatic cancer. And, if that didn't happen, maybe Mrs. Jackson would, as Lennox had said she might, beat the disease herself.

Despite all the progress we've made in the last twenty—or thirty, or fifty—years, we've still barely reached the threshold of truly understanding human beings. To quote Dr. Lewis Thomas, the head of the Sloan Kettering Institute, writing in the June 1978 edition of the *New England Journal of Medicine:* "I am convinced, on nothing more substantial than a strong hunch, that we are, at this stage of our development, a profoundly ignorant species. We have hardly begun to learn. Perhaps already, after only a few centuries of science, we are missing the point, some point or other. Perhaps there is, after all, a point. We have not come to the end of knowledge by a long shot; we have only come to the edge of it."

Gradually, I came out of my slump. So, inevitably, we all die; still, as long as a patient is alive, there's hope. (Even after we die there is, of course, hope, but that's beyond the scope of this book.) Perhaps I'd been too gloomy. Maybe it was the January weather—Minnesota has some terribly long, cold winters, and occasionally they throw me into a slump—but I was going to snap myself out of it and back into what is, really, most of the time, a pretty wonderful world.

So I decided to write about some of the patients I'd treated, or who had been treated by doctors I knew, and who had survived despite long odds against them. We all, now and again, either become ill or have a friend or member of the family who does, and we get depressed. Maybe, I thought, reading about patients who had beaten the odds, survived and thrived when we wise physicians "knew" they couldn't, might give someone who needed it a lift. I know that just reviewing these cases and reliving them mentally has been a stimulating, happy experience for me. I hope it will prove to be as pleasant for the reader.

1

Three-Year-Old Children Are Great Fighters

In August 1972, Helen Roan, then a twenty-seven-year-old teacher married to Ray Roan, an insurance salesman, brought her three-year-old son Jimmy in to see me. I had repaired a hernia on Jimmy when he was eighteen months old and, since no one in the Roan family had been ill since that time, I was the only doctor in Litchfield Helen felt she really knew.

"I'm sorry to bother you with this, Bill," she said, "I know you specialize in surgery and I don't think this is a surgical problem. But you're the doctor we know best so we thought you might not mind if we came to see you first. You can always turn us over to one of your partners."

"I'm glad to see you, Helen—and you too, Jimmy," I said. Jimmy, of course, wasn't paying any attention to me. Helen was holding him and he had his head hung over her shoulder while he sucked his thumb. I looked briefly at his record. "Almost two years since we did that hernia repair, isn't it? I hope he's not still mad at me."

"No," Helen said, smiling, "I'm sure he's forgotten all about that."

"What's bothering him now?" I asked.

"I don't really know," Helen answered. "He's just not himself. Usually when I get home from school he's so glad to see me that he's up and running around like a little demon. He's always laughing and playing with his toys. Lately I've even been thinking perhaps I'd quit teaching, at least until he's in school, so I could spend more time with him. But for the past month all the spark has gone out of him. He naps a lot and doesn't seem to have much energy. All he does is lie around. And it's all I can do to get him to eat.

"There isn't any single thing I can put my finger on," she added. "I just have the feeling something must be wrong with him."

Ordinarily I leave problems like these to my partners; in fact, it's the rare patient who gets to see me unless the complaint is surgical. My partners, and all the nurses and aides who work in our clinic, know how much I dislike general practice. I'm afraid I've many times made that more than apparent.

But Helen Roan is an attractive, pleasant, intelligent woman and I'd enjoyed the few conversations I'd had with her when I had Jimmy in the hospital for his hernia repair. So, rather than referring him immediately to one of my partners, I decided I'd check him over. I wasn't very busy that afternoon anyway.

Jimmy was cooperative while I examined him, surprisingly so for a three year old. Ordinarily children that young yelp and fight if you even try to listen to their hearts. But Jimmy just lay there on the examining table and let me push and prod wherever I wished. He didn't even fight the tongue depressor when I examined his throat; and that, as any doctor will agree, is highly unusual behavior for a child of his age.

The only thing I noticed, other than his apathy, was his color. He seemed to me to be just a bit pale. I asked Helen if she had noticed it, but she hadn't. However, that's not so unusual. If you are close to a person, seeing him or her almost every day, you are apt to overlook gradual changes in appearance. (In 1960, about three months after I moved to Litchfield, I caught hepatitis, an inflammation of the liver that, among other things, turns the patient's skin and—most noticeably—the whites of the eyes, yellow. I had a vague feeling something was wrong. I didn't have my usual energy and the cigars, of which I then smoked about five a day, had begun to taste bad [another symptom of hepatitis; patients lose their taste for smoking]. But neither I, nor my wife, nor any of my partners noticed that the whites of my eyes were turning yellow till a radiologist, who hadn't seen me for three weeks, saw me at the hospital and said, "Hey Bill, what's the matter? Have you got hepatitis?" Then of course, the yellow color became apparent to everyone who knew me.)

Just to be complete I decided to ask the lab technician at our clinic to check Jimmy's hemoglobin and—as long as she would have to stick him with a needle anyway—I decided to get a white blood cell count and a differential (a count of the different types of white cells). I didn't expect any abnormalities, but leukemia is by far the most common form of cancer in children and I decided I might as well rule it out.

While we waited for the results Helen and I talked about movies, books and life in Litchfield. It's funny how unhurried a male doctor can become when he has an attractive woman to talk to, and in about five minutes I had the laboratory results back. As I read them I must have winced because Helen, who was watching me, said, "Bill, is there something wrong?"

I looked over at Jimmy, nonchalantly sucking on a lollipop I had given him, not paying us the slightest attention. "I'm afraid so, Helen," I said. "Jimmy's hemoglobin is down to ten; it should be about fourteen. That's why he's so pale. But worse, the white cells in his blood aren't normal. I don't want to use complicated medical terms but I'll have to in order to explain. Normally Jimmy's white blood count should be about seven or eight thousand cells in each cubic millimeter of blood. About seventy percent of these should be what we call neutrophiles and the other thirty percent should be lymphocytes. But Jimmy's white cell count is eleven thousand—in itself, not too high to be alarming—but unfortunately ninety-five percent of the cells are lymphoblasts. Lymphoblasts are very young lymphocytes.

"Helen, I may as well say it because I know you're thinking it anyway; we'll need more tests but it's almost certain that Jimmy has acute lymphoblastic leukemia. That's the most common kind of leukemia in children." Jimmy was still ignoring us and Helen had accepted the news without flinching, so I went on. "I know you'll want to talk with Ray about this—I'm certain it's as much a shock to you as it is to me—but I think the quicker we get Jimmy on proper treatment the better the results. Would you like to have me call Ray at his office and see if we can get him down here right now? Or would you rather talk it over with him first?"

"If you have the time I'd just as soon get it over with," Helen said. "Jimmy can play with some of the toys out in the waiting room if you think he shouldn't be here."

"He doesn't seem to be paying much attention to us," I said, "but perhaps that's not a bad idea. Maybe it would be best if you call Ray. I'll see my last patient and then, by the time he's here, I'll be free to talk."

Twenty minutes later, with all my other patients gone, Ray and Helen and I sat together in my office. One of our nurses had agreed to keep an eye on Jimmy.

Ray is a big, friendly, ruddy-faced man. He was then thirty years old, three years older than Helen. He is intelligent and outgoing, and he had built, in the four years they'd lived in Litchfield, a very successful insurance business.

How a doctor talks with patients depends on a lot of variables. Some patients prefer to be told only in general what the treatment and prognosis are. Others want to know as much as possible about the situation. Some simply aren't sufficiently educated or intelligent enough to understand the complex medical terminology that is sometimes required to understand a disease and its treatment. Usually, however, if the doctor makes a real effort and explains the specialized terms that can't be avoided, the patient will understand all that's necessary for intelligent participation in treatment of the illness. I knew Ray and Helen could certainly understand and would want to know about the problems they were going to have to face.

"To begin with, Ray, let me tell you that, based on the smear which shows us the cells in Jimmy's blood, there's virtually no doubt that he has leukemia. The kind he has is known as acute lymphoblastic leukemia and it's the most common of all the leukemias in children. In the United States there are about 2000 cases of leukemia discovered in children every year and eighty percent of these are the acute lymphoblastic type. Leukemia is—and I hate to use this word—a form of cancer. It's cancer of the blood.

"Now, let me make it clear at the outset that neither I nor any of my partners will be treating Jimmy. I don't treat leukemia because it's not a surgical disease. My partners don't treat it because the advances in the medical treatment of some cancers have been coming at such a rapid rate that only someone who is involved on a daily basis with this sort of disease can possibly keep in his head the knowledge required to treat it properly. I can almost say without exaggeration that if a doctor hasn't read the most recent issues of the journals that cover advances in the treatment of these diseases, then he may have missed something new and valuable. So, with your permission, I'll refer Jimmy to someone in Minneapolis who specializes in diseases of the blood. If you prefer, I'll send him to the Mayo Clinic. There are specialists there who are expert in treating leukemia. I'll leave that to you."

"If you think they can do the job in Minneapolis, that will probably be easiest for us," Ray said. "Helen's sister lives in the suburbs and she can stay there as long as Jimmy has to be in the hospital. I assume he will have to be, for a while anyway."

"For a while, yes," I said, "but possibly not for more than a week. I'm sure they'll want to get some special X-rays and undoubtedly they'll want a sample of the bone marrow. After that they may decide to give him an initial course of treatment while he's in the hospital, just in case the medicines make him sick. Then you'll probably be able to bring him home and we can give him the medicines he'll need and check his blood periodically. We'll just follow his doctor's instructions. We've done that before.

"Now I'm not going to tell you exactly what drugs they'll prescribe or in what doses because, frankly, I don't know enough about the field to do that. What I can say is that, after the appropriate tests, they'll start him on some rather powerful drugs in order to obtain, if they can, a complete remission of his disease. That is, they'll try to get his blood and bone marrow back to what appears to be a completely normal condition. They can successfully do this in ninety-five percent of patients.

"Then comes the strenuous time for you, Jimmy and all the rest of us. We keep him on some combination of drugs, whatever the hematologist decides is best for the specific type of leukemia Jimmy has, and we watch his blood for any sign of recurrence. If we're lucky, after three to four years we can discontinue all treatment. Then—again, if we're lucky—Jimmy will stay in remission, which is a cautionary way of saying he'll have been cured.

"I can also tell you this; right now we're still learning new things about all tumors, but we're learning very rapidly about leukemia. I can't honestly tell you what the chances are of Jimmy being cured because I don't know what discovery may be made tomorrow. But I can say this. Ten years ago ninety-five percent of children who developed acute lymphoblastic leukemia died of their disease, usually within three years of diagnosis. Now the chances of a cure are far greater and getting better every day. So let's just keep our fingers crossed and get on with the treatment.

"I'm sure questions will come up as time goes on. I can make the initial referral for you and set up an appointment very soon; after that I think it will be better if one of my partners takes over from this end, since they have more experience in managing this sort of case than I do. You decide who you want and I'll tell him about Jimmy's problem. Think it over and you can let me know tomorrow." I looked at my watch. "It's almost quarter to six now," I said, "so it's too late to reach anyone in Minneapolis. I'll call tomorrow and then will call you at about noon, if that's okay, Helen. I'm going to call Dr. Ted Flanders [pseudonym] who I'm sure you'll like."

"That will be fine," she said, "the sooner the better. I'd like to have him start treatment today if he can."

"I know exactly how you feel, Helen. I'd feel the same if it were my child. You can be certain we'll get things moving as fast as possible."

Two days later Jimmy was under the care of a hematologist in Minneapolis. The first few days were rough on Helen and Ray as well as Jimmy. The hospital was one where they treated many children with leukemia and that helped Helen; she had a chance to talk with other mothers who were going through the same anguish. The diagnosis we had made on the blood smear was confirmed when the bone marrow aspiration was done. Jimmy was kept in the hospital for the first two weeks of treatment.

To everyone's delight he responded beautifully. The drugs caused some nausea and he lost most of his hair, but Jimmy was one of the ninety-five percent in whom

the disease went into a complete remission. Two weeks
later he was home, in school, and taking medicines under the supervision of one of my partners, who kept in
touch with the hematologist by phone.

Every couple of months Jimmy went back to Minneapolis for a checkup. He stayed in remission.

During one of our long cold winters, he developed
pneumonia; one of the side effects of some of the anticancer drugs is that they lower the patient's resistance
to disease because, even though they mainly destroy
cancer cells, they also suppress the normal germ-
fighting cells that are produced by the bone marrow.
Fortunately, with all the potent antibiotics we now
have, it's usually possible to cure most infections with
relative ease. We were able to clear up Jimmy's
pneumonia in our own hospital.

In 1976, four years after we had made the diagnosis
of leukemia, Jimmy was still in remission. I met Helen
and Jimmy in the clinic one afternoon, after they had
been to see my partner, and Helen said, "Bill, I'm
almost afraid to do it but Dr. Flanders is going to take
Jimmy off of all medicines. He's been reducing the
doses gradually for the last six months and Jimmy is still
fine. Now he thinks it's safe to discontinue them completely."

"Great, Helen," I said. "I know you'll worry—that's
natural—but even I know enough about what's been
happening in chemotherapy to be certain there's an excellent chance Jimmy is cured. Try to relax and enjoy it.

"Incidentally, Jimmy," I said to him, "wasn't that
you I saw out at the arena the other day skating with one
of the squirt teams? You're going to be quite a hockey
player."

Jimmy, as most children of seven would, just beamed
with pride.

Now it's 1980 and Jimmy is eleven years old. He has
been off all treatment for four years and there is no sign
of a recurrence of his disease. We're always cautious

about using the word "cure" when we talk about cancer, but it seems as if it's an appropriate word to apply to Jimmy. We are all, of course, absolutely delighted that things worked out so well for him. Twenty years ago it was a virtual certainty that he wouldn't have had more than a few months after the diagnosis was made.

We haven't, by a long shot, solved the mystery of leukemia. Until we discover what causes the disease we'll never have a "certain" cure. But in 1980 most doctors who specialize in treating these diseases feel safe in predicting that at least fifty percent of those children who develop acute lymphoblastic leukemia will not only be alive but in complete remission and off all therapy after five years. When you consider that in the 1960's ninety-five percent of these children were doomed, it's apparent that we've made great strides. Now it's a matter of continuing to investigate the disease so that, by 1990, we'll be able to cure them all.

That is not, in the opinion of investigators in the field, an unreasonable expectation.

2

One Day at a Time

On July 20, 1955, Gil Slinden, thirty-eight, who was then a lineman for our rural electric agency, was admitted to the Meeker County Hospital.

One week earlier he had come to the clinic to see one of my partners, Fred Schnell, to tell him that he had "some kind of a lump in my left armpit." Fred gave him a complete physical examination but couldn't find anything abnormal other than what he later described in his operative note as a "walnut-sized" mass in the left axilla (armpit). Fred couldn't tell what it was, since there was no obvious evidence either of tumor or infection that might have drained into a gland in the axilla, so he suggested that Gil come to the hospital so Fred could remove what he suspected was an enlarged lymph node; or, as they are commonly called, lymph gland.

Nodes in the axilla can be deceptively difficult to remove. When you examine the patient it invariably feels as if the gland is lying just beneath the skin but almost always they lie considerably deeper. Assuming the patient is in good health the wise, experienced surgeon will schedule the operation to be done under general anesthesia. Nodes can be removed under local—I know, having done so many times when I was a resident at Bellevue where it was difficult to get operating time—and I can attest to the fact that it is a difficult, bloody, trying experience for the surgeon and almost always a painful one for the patient.

Gil was, and still is, a high-strung patient, which is another good reason for using general anesthesia. "Jumpy" patients aren't good subjects for surgery under local unless the procedure is very minor—say, a wart removal—and even then most surgeons will sedate them fairly heavily preoperatively. In fact, before I go to the dentist, I usually take some sort of tranquilizer; I hate to have my teeth worked on under local or no anesthesia.

On July 20 Gil came in to the hospital at 7:30 A.M. He hadn't eaten since midnight. According to the operative note Fred began operating at 8:21 A.M., and by 8:30 he had the gland out and the wound closed; Fred is a very fast surgeon. He felt that he had removed the entire gland and none of the other twelve or so lymph nodes that are normally in the axilla seemed to be enlarged.

The pathology report, which came back on July 22, described the node as a "malignant lymphoblastoma." The pathologist added, "I believe this is a lymphosarcoma rather than leukemia." Lymphosarcoma is, like leukemia, a type of cancer.

In 1955 we didn't have the wide variety of anticancer drugs that we now have, nor did we have the sophisticated X-ray techniques which sometimes enable us to find tumor involvement in areas we can't see, feel or visualize with conventional X-ray. Fred referred Gil to the Mayo Clinic and they recommended radiation to the left upper chest on the assumption that if there was tumor in one gland there was probably tumor elsewhere in that area. Two years later, when Gil had pain in his spine, he was given a course of nitrogen mustard. Nitrogen mustard was about the only anticancer drug available in 1959 and it was widely used, though usually with little success.

Over the next twelve years Gil didn't develop any more swollen glands or organs, or any other signs of lymphosarcoma, though in the first three years after his operation he did have pains in the arms and legs for which he was given nitrogen mustard therapy on the assumption that they were caused by lymphosarcoma pressing on nerves; whether this was true or not will probably never be known.

From 1959 till 1966 he developed no new lumps. Then, in 1966, a small gland could be felt on his right groin. Fred removed it and the pathologist's report was, again, malignant lymphoma. This time Gil was given a course of treatment with one of the newer anticancer drugs.

Gil had, understandably, become very concerned every time he developed any sign or symptom that suggested he might have a recurrence of the disease. Over the next twelve years he had two more glands removed—one from the area of the elbow, another from the groin—both of which were normal. In a patient without Gil's history the glands probably wouldn't even have been removed.

Gil also developed a bleeding duodenal ulcer, probably from the stress of living with a disease that in most cases would have caused death years earlier. The ulcer was quickly cured with medical treatment and, except for a hernia repair in 1977, Gil had only the usual minor medical problems with which most of us are occasionally plagued. He continued to work at the Rural Electric Office and, in fact, has been the director of the office for several years.

Then, in July 1978, Gil slipped and fell at home, landing on his right scapula ("wing bone"). He didn't think much of it till it began to swell. About a week after the accident, he came to the clinic where Fred saw him and took X-rays which showed a fracture of the scapula. Fred naturally assumed that the swelling in the area was caused by bleeding from the fracture and advised only rest of the shoulder and hot packs to speed resorption of the blood.

After two weeks of this treatment the mass was no smaller; in fact, it seemed larger to both Fred and Gil. Fred asked me to see Gil. The mass felt awfully hard and, with the benefit of the hindsight I had as a result of the two fruitless weeks of treatment, I suspected it might be a tumor. We ordered some special X-rays—a series of X-ray pictures that showed the mass at different depths—and the radiologist now decided that what had first looked like a simple fracture was, in fact, a fracture in a bone invaded by a malignant tumor.

This was not the sort of case for which I wanted to provide the care. Malignant tumors in the scapula are very rare. They can be treated in different ways; surgical removal, X-ray, chemotherapy or a combination of any or all of these. I'd never even heard of a tumor of the scapula, so I decided that this would best be treated at a big medical center to which we doctors who serve small communities send our unusual cases. Since Gil had already been treated once at the Mayo Clinic I referred him back there. The doctor to whom I spoke was understanding. "I imagine Mr. Slinden is very apprehensive," he said, "so I'll squeeze him into my schedule quickly." Two days later Gil was in the Mayo Clinic.

After the usual complete examination a biopsy was scheduled; i.e., a small piece of the tumor was removed and examined under the microscope. It was, once again, a malignant lymphoma. The doctor in charge of Gil's case decided to try X-ray treatment, since it had been almost twenty-three years since he had had X-ray treatment to the right side of his chest. Besides, with the new X-ray therapy machines we now have, it's possible to deliver large doses of X-ray to the tumor without damaging deeper structures—in Gil's case, his lung.

The tumor responded beautifully. It was, when I felt it, almost the size of a grapefruit. Just five months later, I couldn't feel any tumor at all, nor could his doctor at the Mayo Clinic. It's too early to say, of course, but it seems reasonable to hope that Gil is once again "cured" of his malignant lymphoma.

This case exemplifies several things, most of which either are vaguely known or completely unknown to the general public.

First, all cancers aren't the same. If you look up the word "cancer" in a medical dictionary you will find that it comes from the Latin word for crab. Different dictionaries may then expand in different ways but mine (Blakiston's *New Gould Medical Dictionary*) says, "Any malignant tumor including carcinoma and sarcoma; formerly a synonym of carcinoma." Then there are many subdivisions of cancer listed.

Basically, however, cancer falls into two categories, carcinoma and sarcoma. Carcinomas arise in tissue which is classified as epithelial; that is, it is composed of contiguous cells with a minimum of intercellular tissue. It forms the skin and lines hollow organs and all passages of the respiratory, digestive and genitourinary system. Thus most malignant tumors of the skin, intestine, bladder and lung are carcinomas.

Sarcomas arise in tissues classified as nonepithelial such as bone, muscle and lymph nodes.

Both sarcomas and carcinomas can invade the lymphatic system and/or the bloodstream and spread to other organs.

For all practical purposes the lay person may just as well classify all malignant tumors as cancers, but—and this is very important—he or she should understand that not all cancers behave the same. Some grow slowly and almost never spread to other organs. Some grow rapidly and spread quickly. Though tumors in individuals may behave in different ways it is safe to say that most cancers of the same classification will tend to behave the same way, slow or aggressive, in afflicted patients. But the exceptions to this rule are so many—as we shall see—that it is barely a rule at all.

Now, back to Gil.

It is now twenty-three years since Gil's diagnosis was made and he still lives a full life. We'll have to suspect that there are still tumor cells in Gil's body—after all, they have been reappearing periodically for almost a quarter century—but they always seem to respond quickly to treatment. Gil's body has obviously acquired some tolerance for these malignant cells. Other cells in Gil's body probably act to kill off or at least to limit the spread of his lymphoma cells. We don't know how this works, how to identify this fighting power, but Gil's life is proof that it exists.

Finally—and this point is only minimally related to Gil's unusual case—we have, over the last twenty-five years, made great strides in treating certain kinds of cancer; the treatment of lymphomas and leukemias is one of the fields of therapy that has advanced most. Now, using combinations of recently developed anticancer drugs, it's the rare patient who can't be kept alive for several years. Some have even been cured; i.e., they have lived for more than five years without receiving any anticancer drugs. Our cure rates for breast, lung and bowel cancer haven't improved greatly—though, as we'll see in another case, even some of these patients follow unpredictable courses—but in the blood and lymph gland cancers we've made great strides.

Gil Slinden has to be classified as a lucky man. He developed a malignant disease in the years before we had the sophisticated treatment methods we now have and still he has been able to live a full, rewarding life.

This is probably as satisfactory a place as any to mention the problem of the patient who has had cancer and goes on to live for weeks, months or years. There is little doubt that, at least for the first few months after their treatment, many will probably be very wary of any symptom they develop. A bad cold will send them flying to the doctor for reassurance that it is a cold and not cancer that has spread to the lung. On the other hand, some patients seem to be able to forget about their surgical, drug and/or radiation treatment as soon as it's completed.

How the individual will react to his or her experience with cancer treatment will depend partly on the type of cancer they had, partly on the moral support the doctor gives them, but mostly on the personality and age of the individual who has had the disease. Nervous people are going to be easily alarmed at any deviation from the normal; phlegmatic people are going to live as calmly as if they'd simply had a touch of the flu.

As far as how the doctor should deal with his post-cancer-treatment patient, there is only one generalization possible; be honest. If I think my patient has been cured, I tell her so. If I think she is likely to have a recurrence in a few months or a year, I'll say something like, "As far as I can tell you are now cured. I'd advise you to go out and live one day at a time. If trouble returns we'll fight it, but it may never return and there's no sense spoiling your life by worrying about something that may never happen."

For those patients whose cancer I've been unable to cure—say, for example, a woman with breast cancer which has recurred in her spine—I paint the most optimistic reasonable picture possible. I tell her that there are still many things we can do to control and slow down the growth of the cancer. I tell her of the constant research that is continuing into its cause and treatment. And I tell her, finally, that there is no case any doctor can label as hopeless; often patients get better even when we expect that they won't.

The whole problem of how to manage the patient who has had cancer is too extensive for a thorough discussion here. I'd summarize it by saying that with continuing physical and moral support from family, doctor, and friends, most people can continue to live productive, happy lives after fighting the cancer battle.

They wouldn't be normal if they weren't occasionally worried that the disease might recur but, particularly with the passage of time, such concerns occur less frequently.

Taking life a day at a time is, in fact, the only sensible approach for anyone, cancer victim or not. It's a rule I try—not always successfully—to follow.

3

Riding the Tiger

When I was at Bellevue, between 1953 and 1960, there were surgeons here and there across the country doing what came to be known as the "super-radical" mastectomy. In patients who had cancer of the breast the surgeon would not only remove the breast, the underlying muscles of the chest wall and all the contents of the axilla, which was the then "standard" radical mastectomy; they would also open the chest along the sternum (breast bone) and remove the glands that run along the inside of the chest in this area. Their theory was that, since some cancers spread not only to the lymph glands in the axilla but to the glands beneath the sternum, they would save a few patients who might otherwise die of cancer by removing these glands.

I suppose it's possible that they did save a few patients with this super-radical procedure, but in general the operation was a colossal flop. The number of people killed by extending the operation was far greater than the number the operation saved. I vividly remember one Monday evening when I was chief resident, making rounds with the director of our surgical service and all the interns and assistant residents, and asking him, after we had just discussed a patient with breast cancer and were out of her hearing range, "Dr. Stevens, what do you think of the super-radical mastectomy? Do you think perhaps we ought to start doing them on our patients?''

"Bill," he said, "it's a shame that the surgeons who are doing this operation haven't read any surgical history. If they had, they'd know that Dr. Bloodgood tried the same procedure years ago and it was a disaster. There's an aphorism that almost applies here, 'Don't be first with the latest.' Only in this instance they seem to think they're being first with something already decades old. Stay away from the super-radical mastectomy. In another year or so only those who are too stubborn to confess their errors will be doing the procedure.''

And that's the way it worked out. Even now, in 1980, there are still some doctors, mostly in major cancer treatment centers, who do this procedure. Why, only they and God know. It certainly isn't because they've been able to prove that they're saving any lives.

In 1980, in fact, the number of surgeons who perform even the standard radical mastectomies for breast cancer has diminished markedly. The reports from virtually every surgical center in the world show that the modified radical mastectomy in which the breast and the axillary contents (fat and lymph nodes) are removed, produces just as high a cure rate as does the "radical" mastectomy, in which the muscles of the chest wall are also removed. And the modified radical is cosmetically and functionally superior to the radical. It also causes fewer complications. In particular, it is less likely to cause the chronic swelling of the arm that is seen in about fifteen percent of patients who have undergone the radical procedure.

In 1968, however, most surgeons were still routinely doing radical mastectomies for breast cancer. Routine procedure in women with breast lumps was to put them to sleep with a general anesthetic, perform a biopsy (remove either the entire lump, if it was small, or a piece of it, if it was large), have the pathologist examine it under the microscope and then, if the biopsy showed can-

cer, go ahead with the radical mastectomy. Only a few
surgeons in the United States, foremost among them
Dr. George Crile of Cleveland, were risking not only
malpractice suits but the wrath of their fellow surgeons
by performing modified radical mastectomies or even
partial mastectomies (the so-called "lumpectomy," in
which only the lump and a margin of normal breast
tissue are removed) in selected cases. It wasn't until
about 1971 that these less radical procedures began to
achieve acceptance by the medical profession; and, as
I've already noted, there are still surgeons who swear,
despite all the evidence to the contrary, that the
traditional radical mastectomy (popularized by Dr.
William Halsted in a paper published in 1894) is the only
acceptable method for treating breast cancer. Traditional methods die hard. It's understandably difficult
for a surgeon to concede that for years he had been
routinely performing an operation more radical than
necessary.

However, in 1969, when Flora Lewis came in to see
me, I was still performing the traditional radical mastectomy. (In 1969 I didn't know any better. Since 1971 I
have done a radical mastectomy only once, in 1976, and
that was on a woman whose family had close ties to
Memorial Hospital in New York City where, at that
time, the radical mastectomy still reigned supreme. I explained to her I felt the radical operation was unnecessary but, at her insistence, I reluctantly proceeded.
Perhaps I should have refused, but she needed a breast
cancer operation, and the choices were a radical or no
operation at all.)

Flora was forty-one in 1969. She owns and manages a
clothing store for women in a town near Litchfield; she
lives in Litchfield because her husband, Jim, owns a
grocery store in town. Flora plays bridge a lot and, according to my wife, Joan, who plays in a bridge club
with her, is one of the best players in town.

I have always enjoyed talking with Flora when we

meet at parties, as we often do, because Flora is extremely intelligent, an ardent Republican who reads about and understands political issues and loves to discuss them. I am about ninety percent Democrat and Flora and I often get into heated arguments, particularly around election time. I have to concede that most of my political expertise is pure bluff; I can't get away with that when arguing with Flora. I always learn something from her, even though she can't often persuade me to change my voting plans.

Flora and Jim have two sons, the same ages as two of our boys, and their children often visit at our home. And of course having children of about the same age gives us something else to talk about when we meet. One of the things about which Flora and I agree is that our children are involved in far too many extracurricular activities; we are both sick of going to evening music concerts and athletic events. But, dutiful parents that we are, we continue to go. Joan and I have always enjoyed Flora and Jim's company. For that reason I was particularly distressed to find that Flora had a large, almost certainly malignant, breast lump.

"I've got a lump on my left breast, Bill," she told me. "I've known about it for six months and I've been praying it would go away, but it doesn't look as if it will. In fact, it seems to be getting bigger and now I think I can feel another small lump in my armpit."

You would think, with all the publicity breast cancer gets, stories like Flora's would be rare, but they aren't. Many patients practice self-denial when they have symptoms that may suggest cancer (the famous "seven signs" the cancer authorities publicize), but women with breast lumps are the most notorious self-deluders of all. I understand why—they don't want to admit they have a sign or symptom which may eventually lead to the loss of a breast—and I consider this one reason why we doctors should emphasize that the earlier a lump is found, the better the chance the patient may be cured by a conservative operation, perhaps without even removing the breast.

As far as Flora was concerned it was too late for such philosophizing. I may tell a husband that I wish his wife had come to the office sooner; I never say that to the patient. She knows only too well that the delay may be costly, but there isn't any way to turn the clock back so I don't belabor this distressing fact. In fact, I often tell her that the delay may not have reduced her chances of cure anyway. Actually this may be true. Some reported series of cases suggest that the chances of curing at least some patients aren't affected at all by delays between discovery of a lump and its treatment; though it would seem only logical, and is probably true in many cases, that the sooner the proper treatment is applied to a breast cancer, the better a woman's chance of being cured.

Flora's lump had all the classic signs of cancer. It was hard; it had caused the nipple to invert and there were at least two small, firm lymph nodes that I could feel in the axilla. I ordered mammograms of both breasts. The X-rays of the right breast, which had felt normal, showed no suspicious signs; on the X-rays of the left breast could be seen what appeared to be a cancer.

After I'd talked the situation over with Flora and Jim, they elected to have me proceed with the radical mastectomy if the biopsy was positive. Nowadays many women choose to "wait and decide later"; they'd prefer to make one decision at a time and to go to sleep knowing that, whether or not the lump is cancer, they'll still have their breast when they wake up. Flora preferred to avoid a second anesthetic. Besides, in her case I was virtually certain the lump was malignant, and told her so.

It was and so, after I had the biopsy report, I proceeded to do the radical mastectomy. The final report from the pathologist showed an "infiltrating ductal carcinoma with metastasis in seven of thirteen lymph nodes.''

This pathology report, when it came back on the fifth postoperative day, was not very encouraging. Actually, sad to say, even with all our educational campaigns, X-rays and new drugs, the overall mortality, if we consider all breast cancer cases, is about the same as it was sixty years ago. Our cure rate is about seventy percent. But in cases like Flora's, with extensive involvement outside the breast itself, the cure rate from surgery, even with radiation therapy, is only about twenty percent. (Since these relatively advanced cases are included in the overall statistics, it should be clear that the woman with an early case, confined to the breast, has about an eighty-five percent chance of being cured.)

I didn't tell Flora and Jim these statistics. There was nothing to be gained by it. If they had asked me for a prognosis I would have given them the figures, but I'd have emphasized a point a surgical mentor of mine often made during my training period. When we residents would cite percentages, mostly to show off our erudition, he'd say, ''Don't bother me with statistics; it's a hundred percent for the person who has it.'' I'd have emphasized that Flora might well be among the twenty percent cured and that there was nothing to be gained by dwelling on the possibility that she wasn't.

Flora and Jim took the news well. I always emphasize the positive—in this case, the fact that patients with disease in the same stage as Flora's could be cured—and I arranged X-ray treatment for her. I referred her to Willmar, a town thirty-five miles from Litchfield, where the radiologists used cobalt therapy and treated the axilla, the area above the clavicle (collar bone), and the portion of her chest behind the sternum. These are the areas which contain lymph nodes to which breast cancer is most likely to spread. Our hope was, of course, that no cancer cells had reached these areas but, if only a few had, there was a possibility, at least, that X-ray treatment would destroy them.

I saw Flora in my office first at three-month intervals, then at six-month intervals, over the next three years. On each visit I'd not only examine her but I'd get a chest X-ray and there was never any evidence of cancer. As we reached the four-year mark we were both hopeful. In treating most cancer we generally speak of "five-year cures," assuming that if the disease hasn't manifested itself in that period of time, then it probably has been cured. With most cancers this is generally true. Unfortunately a few cancers, including breast cancer, may recur after ten or even more years. It may be that these are not recurrences, but entirely new cancers, though the evidence suggests that they are most likely the former rather than the latter.

Unfortunately, when Flora came to my office in June of 1973, exactly four years after her radical mastectomy, she told me, "I've been feeling a little weak, Bill. No pain and no specific problem. I just get tired easily." I checked her hemoglobin level and it was 9.0 grams; 14.0 grams/100 cubic centimeters of blood is normal. Her chest X-ray was normal but when I examined her I could feel her liver. It was enlarged, hard and irregular. After she was dressed I spoke to Flora and Jim, who had driven her into town from their farm about six miles out of town. "I hate to tell you this," I said, "but there isn't any sense in pretending. You're anemic, Flora, and I think it's because the tumor has returned. When I press on your liver it seems to me that I can feel some hard lumps that weren't there before. I'd like to admit you to the hospital. Then we can get some more studies, including X-rays of your liver, that will show whether or not I'm right.

"And remember, even if I am right, there are things we can do. First, we can get your blood level up with iron, liver shots and transfusions, if necessary, so you won't feel tired. Second, we can give you one of the an-

ticancer drugs. Some tumors are very sensitive to them.
You may be one of the lucky ones with that sort of
tumor. We aren't giving up yet—not by a long shot. It's
four years since your mastectomy and you've done very
nicely. We'll do all we can to give you many more good
years."

Flora came into the hospital the next day. She was
forty-five then, and her children, who were sixteen,
fourteen and twelve when she had her breast operation,
were now almost adults. We included them in all the
family discussions.

After getting the basic laboratory work I ordered a
liver scan, a procedure in which a radioactive material is
injected into the patient and picked up by the liver,
enabling us to get X-rays which show the liver in great
detail. The report was depressing to say the least. It
showed "extensive replacement of the right lobe of the
liver [by tumor] and the left lobe shows massive hyper-
trophy [increase in size] which is not uniform in its
lower portion and may, in fact, be partly replaced. The
findings are strongly suggestive of neoplastic [tumor]
replacement of the liver, probably from the patient's
clinically known breast carcinoma."

(Perhaps this is a good place to mention the entire
business of "scanning." When we "scan" a patient,
looking for diseases of the internal organs which may
not be visible on X-ray, we inject into the patient a substance which is ordinarily concentrated in the organ in
which we are interested. We add onto, or "tag," this
substance with radioactive materials. After the injection, X-rays are taken and the radioactive tag will
produce a shadow on the X-ray film. If there is no
radioactive substance in a portion of the organ where we
could expect it to be, then that suggests the organ is
malfunctioning or, as in Flora's case, probably replaced
by tumor tissue.

"Scanning" began, on a practical scale, in 1951 when
radioactive iodine was used to scan the thyroid. In the

1950's radioactive "tags" were developed which enabled us to scan the liver and brain. In 1980 we can and do scan the lung, bone and even the heart, when such scanning is necessary to get information we think will be useful and cannot obtain in any other way. With the development in the late 1960's of X-ray machines that enable us to take three-dimensional X-rays of most parts of the body—the so-called combined axial tomography scanners (or CAT scanners)—the use of radioactive substance injections is not as common as it once was. However, in certain cases such radioactive scanning will still give us information that CAT scanners cannot provide.)

I told Flora and Jim what the liver scan had shown and then told them that, if they agreed, I'd first transfuse Flora with two or three pints of blood and then I wanted to get a liver biopsy to make certain the radiologist was right. After all, the best he could say was "the findings are strongly suggestive." A liver biopsy, which could be done under local anesthesia using a special needle to remove a small cone of liver tissue, would probably give us a certain diagnosis.

Flora agreed to the biopsy and it was done the next day. The report was "metastatic poorly differentiated adenocarcinoma to liver." Now the bad news had been certified.

I then proposed to Flora and Jim that I call a specialist in the use of anticancer drugs and treat Flora as he suggested. They agreed with my plan.

Over the next two days we gave Flora three pints of blood, which brought her hemoglobin level up to normal and made her feel much stronger, and then, after consulting with a chemotherapist, I started her on 5 Fluorouracil, or 5-F-U, one of the most widely used of the anticancer drugs. I kept her in the hospital for the first week, while she received daily injections of the drug, so that we could watch for side effects; as you'll recall from Jimmy Roan's experience, the anticancer drugs, unfortunately, attack normal cells as well as tumor cells. Hopefully, since tumors are usually composed of very rapidly growing cells, the drug will proportionately kill many tumor cells while leaving healthy cells relatively unscathed. But, during the first trial of any anticancer drug, it's best to keep a close watch on the patient, so that if side effects occur secondary to healthy-cell damage, they'll be spotted early.

Flora tolerated the first series of treatments nicely. Her bone marrow, one of the areas most sensitive to anticancer drugs, remained healthy and she didn't develop the nausea or sores in the mouth that occasionally occur when 5-F-U is administered.

She went home after a week of treatment and, a month later, came back into the hospital for another intensive course of therapy. When I saw her in my office, a month after this second treatment, she felt fine again. And, admittedly to my amazement—I'd hoped for a good result but wasn't overly optimistic—her liver was now about normal in size. I could just barely feel it on examination.

"Flora," I said, "you've obviously had an excellent response to the drug; I can't feel any tumor at all in your liver."

"That's wonderful, Bill," she said, "and the injections haven't made me the least bit ill. I'm going to try to just go on living as I have been. I know I'll have days when I get down, but with the store, the kids and Jim to keep me busy I think I'll be able to keep from dwelling on this darn tumor. I'm certainly going to try."

For the last six years we've kept Flora on 5-F-U; one injection a week, given after checking her blood level, and to the great delight of all of us, there has been no evidence of tumor recurrence. Flora knows as well as I do that this could happen. She's grateful for every day of her reprieve, but it has now been ten years since we removed her breast and cancer-infiltrated lymph nodes, and six years since she has been on chemotherapy, and she is clinically well. Maybe we could discontinue the 5-F-U; it's possible that it has killed all the recurrent cancer, but neither she nor I are ready to do so. She's not having any difficulty tolerating the drug and it's as if we're riding a tiger; we're both afraid to have her step off. She's had ten good years despite an extensive tumor with recurrence; I hope she has thirty more.

She has, as we both expected she would, had some days when she gets depressed. I told her when we started drug treatment to call whenever she felt the need to talk to me. Usually, in just a few minutes, I can reassure her that things are going well. Now, when I happen to meet her when she's at the clinic for an injection, she rarely mentions her medical problem. Instead we talk about our children or argue politics as we did in the old days. Emotionally and socially she's apparently just as she was before she ever developed the tumor. If she still has "down" moments, and I suspect she does, she keeps them to herself. Jim told me that she seems just as spirited and cheerful as she was ten years ago, and he certainly ought to know.

I don't want to suggest that every patient with breast cancer will do as well on 5-F-U or any other drug (we'll use another one if she gets a second recurrence) as Flora has done. Some don't benefit at all; some get only transient benefit; a few do as well as Flora. The point is that those few flourish and that, with new anticancer drugs being developed every year, to say nothing (yet) of the drug combinations which are being used, it's possible, even probable, we'll have more patients who, like Flora, if they don't "beat" cancer the first time around, may do so the second or even the third time. It's getting increasingly important that both doctor and patient not give up the fight unless there's absolute evidence that it's pointless to continue the war.

4

Talk About Tough!

Anyone who would like to meet Elizabeth "Bucky" Ryan need only come to Litchfield and call her either at her home or at the Gloria Dei Manor, a nursing home where she has worked part-time since 1977. In 1975 she had to retire as an operating room nurse because she was sixty-five. (Bucky forgives me for revealing her age.) Bucky has been an O.R. nurse since 1948—almost thirty years.

When I arrived in Litchfield in 1960 I immediately became Chief of Surgery at the Meeker County Memorial Hospital. (It has been suggested that I was appointed to this position because I was, and am, the only surgeon on the staff of the Meeker County Hospital. There may be a kernel of truth in this. In any case, I have held the position continuously since my arrival here.)

I met Bucky in the operating room, the Monday after Joan and I and our six children arrived after a long (My God, how long!) drive from New York City where I had, on June 30, 1960, completed my surgical residency at Bellevue Hospital. Bucky is 5'5" and she weighs 93 pounds, the same weight she was back in 1960. She is an excellent operating room nurse and I enjoyed working with her for the next sixteen years. I'm not the sort of temperamental surgeon who throws instruments—that species, thank heavens, is virtually extinct—but I am, occasionally, a trifle grumpy when I first arrive in the hospital operating room at eight in the morning. Not very grumpy, but a little. I shake it off after the first few minutes. The nurses know this and, they've told Joan, they just laugh a little behind my back till I calm down.

Bucky and I worked well together from the very beginning. She was one of those O.R. nurses who always kept an eye on the operation and anticipated just what instrument or suture the surgeon would need next. We never lost any time because Bucky didn't have the proper needle threaded or had forgotten to put a crucial instrument in the sterilizer.

In 1950, Bucky had had a mastectomy for breast cancer. It was another instance where the patient procrastinated a while before going to the doctor (yes, nurses, like other women, do that occasionally), but in Bucky's case the doctor to whom she had finally gone also procrastinated. He thought she had a cyst and that it wasn't unreasonable to watch it for a while, a policy doctors not infrequently follow.

Unfortunately, there was a misunderstanding—a mix-up in communications—and it wasn't till two years after the lump first appeared that the decision was reached to operate and find out whether or not it was a cancer. By that time it had grown from the size of a pea to the size of a marble.

In the days before I moved to Litchfield the G.P.s did some surgery, as they still do, but for major cases a surgeon would drive out from Minneapolis to operate. Bucky, however, preferred to have "her" doctor, Dr. Harold Wilmot, who was an excellent G.P. surgeon, operate on her.

On microscopic examination the tumor proved to be a cancer. Harold did a radical mastectomy, which was the standard procedure for cancer in 1950, and, happily, all the lymph nodes in her armpit were free of tumor. In 1960 ten years had elapsed since her radical mastectomy and it seemed likely that she was cured. In 1979, with Bucky as spritely as ever ("spritely" is a word I rarely use, but it's the perfect word to describe Bucky), it's obvious that her breast cancer was cured despite the delay in surgery.

Then, in 1968, Bucky began to have trouble with constipation. It bothered her for several months but again, she was reluctant to admit that anything might be seriously wrong. She took laxatives as she needed them and waited for her "bowel problem" to clear up. When, after several months, it hadn't, she went to Harold, her family doctor, only after delaying an extra three weeks so she could go to a University of Minnesota football game, an annual outing she had with her son and his family. Harold, knowing Bucky's tendency to put things off, immediately did a proctoscopy, which showed that there wasn't any tumor in the lower ten inches of the large intestine, but the barium enema—an X-ray examination of the colon—showed almost complete obstruction in the sigmoid colon, the portion of the large bowel just above the rectum. He asked me to see her and I agreed with the radiologist's diagnosis of cancer. We gave Bucky laxatives, enemas and an antibiotic which partially sterilizes the bowel and on November 18, 1968, we operated. Before the operation Bucky had said to me, "You won't need to do a colostomy, will you, Dr. Nolen? I'd certainly prefer not to have one." (A colostomy is an operation in which the large intestine is brought out onto the abdominal wall so that stool, which can't get by the obstructing tumor, can empty into a plastic bag. Sometimes a colostomy is permanent; when, for example, the cancerous rectum has to be removed. Sometimes it is done as a temporary measure, for example, when the surgeon thinks his anastomosis [the point where he has sewed the two ends of the bowel together] is a bit insecure and he wants to let it rest while healing. In the case of temporary colostomies, the bowel is usually closed and natural continuity is restored a few weeks later. For obvious reasons patients don't like the idea of colostomies. In fact, once the patient gets used to it, a colostomy is a minor inconvenience. I have many patients who have had them for several years. When they come in for "checkups" they rarely even mention their colostomies.)

I virtually promised Bucky she wouldn't need a colostomy. The tumor was high enough up from the rectum so I was relatively certain I could remove the tumor-containing portion of bowel and sew the upper and lower ends together with ease. And I was afraid that if I said a colostomy was a possibility she would have gone home.

Much to my dismay when I opened Bucky's abdomen, her large intestine was solidly packed with stool. I hadn't realized that the obstruction was so complete that neither laxatives nor enemas had cleaned her out.

"Damn," I said to Fred Schnell, one of my G.P. partners who was assisting me. "This is awful. What I really ought to do is a colostomy. Then we can clean this bowel out through the colostomy, reoperate in a couple of weeks and remove the cancer. The only problem is that I just about promised Bucky I wouldn't do a colostomy. She'll shoot me if I do one. Do you know what she told me to explain waiting for that damn game? She said, 'I figured if I died during the operation, I'd have hated to have missed the game too.' Crazy, but who knows? It makes a sort of sense.

"And, of course," I said, as I reached up and felt the liver, "there isn't any obvious spread now. Maybe a three-week delay will give the damn thing a chance to grow. It feels like it's ready to break through the bowel wall now.

"What do you think I ought to do?"

"You're the surgeon," Fred said, laughing. That's the standard answer when there's a tricky decision to make. And, of course, it's absolutely true. In the O.R. the buck stops with the surgeon.

I thought about it for another couple of minutes while I felt all around the abdomen to make certain there weren't any enlarged glands. Finally I couldn't stall anymore. "Let's get it out," I said. "Just pray we don't get too much spillage."

If you're to understand the rest of Bucky's story I'll have to explain as briefly as I can, trying not to get too technical, how bowel surgery for cancer is done.

First, the surgeon has to free the intestine (intestine is a synonym for "bowel") from any attachments to the back wall of the abdomen. I did this with relative ease.

Next the surgeon decides where he is going to cut across the intestine both above and below the tumor. The places chosen depend on the lymph nodes, the blood supply and other anatomical matters that the reader can ignore. When he has chosen the appropriate points for cutting, where possible taking several inches of normal bowel both above and below the tumor, he places clamps across the bowel at those two places and then cuts out and removes the tumor-containing intestine that lies between the clamps. Finally, he sews the upper and lower ends together, re-forming the hollow tube which is the normal shape of the intestine. Sometimes he can do this using a technique that is called "closed" and, hopefully, allows only tiny amounts of stool to spill; none, if the bowel has been properly prepared. But when one end of the intestine is much wider than the other, he has to use an "open" technique to properly match the two ends. In Bucky's case the upper bowel was markedly distended because of the obstructing tumor; the lower bowel, through which very little stool had passed for several weeks, was almost collapsed. I had to use an open technique to suture the bowel ends together.

I used every trick I know to prevent stool from spilling into the pelvis, but it was all in vain. When I took the clamp off the upper end of the bowel, stool poured into Bucky's abdomen so fast that no matter how vigorously we mopped and used our suction we couldn't begin to keep up with it. Finally, of course, the flood ended, but not before her abdomen was so extensively soiled that even after all the washing we did—and we used several quarts of salt solution (water containing salt of the same concentration as the blood is used to wash out body cavities)—the pelvis was still a fairly dark brown.

"What do you think, Fred?" I asked, knowing very well there wasn't anything more to do.

"I suggest we get out of here," he said, "I'd stick in a couple of drains and close up. There's no doubt she's going to be awfully sick, and we'll probably have to drain a couple of abscesses, but we've done all we can for now."

I agreed. I thought, even then, that perhaps I ought to do a colostomy just in case the suture line broke down. But the line felt secure and a colostomy wasn't going to undo the damage already done.

So we closed. I put a couple of flat, one-inch wide rubber drains in the pelvis in the remote possibility that if an abscess did begin to form it would ooze out along these rubber drains, and then we closed the abdomen.

When Bucky was back in the recovery room I went to speak to her daughter Mary, a nurse, and her son John, a dentist. I told them what had happened. "I'm sorry as the devil," I said. "I should never have promised her I wouldn't do a preliminary colostomy. If I had gotten X-rays today I'd have probably seen she was packed with stool, but after all the laxatives and enemas I was certain she'd be cleaned out. I'm afraid she's in for a stormy postoperative course. The least we can expect is a bad wound infection. We'll just have to wait and see."

"Oh, Dr. Nolen," Mary said, "You ought to know Mom better than that after all this time. She's small but she's tough. She'll be all right. Besides, I went to Mass for her this morning."

"I'm glad to hear that," I said, "We need all the help we can get. And don't worry. I'll keep a close eye on her."

"I know you will," Mary said, "Mom has a lot of faith in you." *That*, I thought, *only shows how poor someone's judgment can be.*

So we watched and waited. First day, a low-grade temperature, only up to 100°, about what I expect with any operation. Second day, still no problems; hardly a drop of drainage from the drains and Bucky was up in a chair. Third day, I listened to her abdomen with my stethoscope and, to my great delight, I heard bowel sounds; her intestines were beginning to function. "Dr. Nolen," Bucky said, "can't you get this tube out and give me something to eat? And stop looking so glum, I'm going to be fine." (Like most surgeons I pass a hollow rubber or plastic tube about ¼" in diameter through the nose into the stomach to put the stomach and intestine at rest till the bowel starts working again after surgery. This tube is usually referred to as a Levin tube, named after the doctor who first thought of using it.)

"Tell you what, Bucky," I said. "As soon as you pass gas from your rectum (a sign the bowel is open and working) I'll take the tube out."

"I passed some this morning," she said. "Now get this darn thing out."

I pulled it out and ordered a liquid diet. I had already pulled the drains out part way—they had never drained anything—and by the fifth postoperative day they were completely out, Bucky was eating a regular diet and walking up and down the halls. She had never run a temperature above 100°.

"Fred," I said, when I discharged Bucky to her home, "this has got to be some kind of miracle. I was about as certain as you can be that we'd all but killed her in the O.R."

Fred laughed and agreed. "Frankly," he said, "I've never seen so much stool in anyone's abdomen as we had in Bucky's. It's amazing she made it."

Six weeks later Bucky was back at work, chipper as ever. I'd told her how the operation had gone—after all, her co-workers in the O.R. knew, and, besides, you can't keep secrets in a small hospital—but she just laughed.

"I knew I'd be all right, Dr. Nolen," she said. "I knew you'd cure me."

Well, I certainly hadn't known I would. And, though I played a role in her recovery, I'm still not certain why she survived. I hesitate to call it a miracle, but it's darn near in that class. Bucky's faith in me; her daughter's, and Bucky's, faith in the Lord; a determination to live; and a rugged constitution all helped Bucky make it.

Tonight I'm going out to our local golf club—there's a farewell dinner for our operating room supervisor—and I'm sure Bucky will be there. We'll have a couple of chuckles over her operation. But, deep down, I know she, like me, realizes that some extraordinary forces helped her to survive.

We are both grateful for that help.

5

Don't Pick the Doctor Who
Got Straight A's—
Pick the One Who'll
Get Up at Night

On the night of May 15, 1974, the phone near
my bed rang at 12:15. Usually I go to bed about 10:30 or
11:00, so I was sleeping soundly when it rang, but I was
fully awake and alert the moment I picked up the
receiver. After practicing medicine for twenty-seven
years (it was twenty-one years, back in 1974), you learn
to get all your faculties functioning efficiently in a very
few seconds, even when roused from a deep sleep.

"Dr. Nolen," I said, answering the phone.

"Bill, this is Lennox." Lennox Danielson is, as I've
mentioned, one of the G.P.s who practices in Litchfield.
"I've got a fellow over here who is sicker than the devil
and I think he's got a surgical problem. Can you come
over and take a look at him?"

"Sure," I answered, "I'll be right there." Joan slept
through the conversation.

I got up, went to the living room, where I always leave
my clothes at night so I can dress without disturbing
Joan, and about ten minutes after Lennox's call I was at
the hospital.

The Meeker County Hospital is located on the south

side of town, on the main street that runs through
Litchfield. From seven in the morning till nine at night
it's a very busy place—patients arriving in cars or by
ambulance, technicians scuttling around drawing blood
and wheeling patients to X-ray, the operating room
almost always busy with one patient being wheeled in
and/or another wheeled out. All the staff doctors have
their cars parked in the small "doctors' " lot at the
north end of the building; in the bigger lots on the south
and west sides are the cars of the people who work in the
kitchen, the laundry and in administration. It's an active, bustling place.

But at night the entire scene changes. If there are any
doctors there, their cars are parked on the south side at
the visitors' entrance; all other entrances are locked at
9:00 P.M., after the last visitors leave. Lights shine in the
entryway, where a receptionist is on duty all night, and
at the nurses' stations on each of the floors. There may
also be a light visible in a private room of a patient with
insomnia. Otherwise the hospital, like most of the
patients, is at rest. As I drove up to the visitors' entrance
I noticed the cars of the night duty nurses—perhaps half
a dozen in a lot that would contain fifty during the
day—and Lennox's car. I entered the quiet hospital and
was told by the receptionist that Dr. Danielson and his
patient were in X-ray. I walked down the flight of stairs
to our basement X-ray department.

Lennox met me in the corridor outside the X-ray
rooms. "I've never seen this patient before," Lennox
said. "His name is Tommy French and he lives in
Walnut Grove, where he works as a carpenter. He's
twenty-eight years old. I came over here at eleven-thirty
to see a patient of mine with a coronary and as I was
parking my car this fellow's girl friend asked me if I'd
see him. He was standing by his car in the visitors'
parking lot with the dry heaves. I got a wheel chair and
we brought him into Emergency. I listened to their story

and examined him and then thought I'd better call you."

Lennox, as you may have noted, hadn't yet told me what he thought the diagnosis was. Often, when we ask another doctor to consult on a patient, that's a little game we play; we don't tell the consultant what we think the diagnosis is because we don't want to influence his own appraisal. Naturally, if the patient has been in the hospital for a few days or weeks, as the consultant reviews the chart he's going to read what diagnosis the doctor has been considering, but with newly admitted patients there is no record to see.

"Before you talk to him," Lennox said, "let me brief you on his history. I got most of it from his girl friend, who's upstairs filling out the admission forms.

"According to her, and she seems reliable, this Tommy has been living like a wild man for the last year. He's a hard worker but with the building slump he's had trouble finding work. When he doesn't have a job he sits around and drinks coffee and smokes cigarettes all day. Then he gets hyped up and he hits the local taverns. He hasn't been eating anything but candy bars for about a month. She tells me he's been complaining of vague stomachaches for the last couple of weeks. She tries to get him to eat, but he won't—when you see him you'll see how skinny he is—just candy bars, coffee and beer.

"This afternoon at about four o'clock, his stomach pains suddenly got worse and he had to take the last hour off from work. He's got a temporary job with another carpenter building a house just outside of Walnut Grove. He came home and took a couple of aspirin but he couldn't keep them down. In fact, he couldn't keep anything down—milk, soup, not even water. The pain finally got so bad his girl friend persuaded him to go to see the doctor in Walnut Grove. I don't know if you know that guy, but I do. He's a lazy son of a gun who shouldn't even be practicing medicine.

"Anyway, they drove right to the doctor's office, which is in his home. He came to the door, they told him about the pain, and he told them to go home, go to bed, and come back in the morning. Didn't even examine Tommy. Hard to believe, isn't it?" I nodded in agreement.

"It was almost eleven by then and the girl, her name is Ruth, decided Tommy was too sick to go home. She got him in the car and drove the forty miles here, going like the devil. She'd arrived just a few seconds before I drove into the lot. That's about all there is to the story. Why don't you go in and see him; they must be done taking X-rays by now."

I walked into the X-ray room and saw Tommy French stretched out on the table. He was clearly miserable. His eyes were sunken, he was pale and sweaty, there was vomitus drooling from the corner of his mouth. He looked like he hadn't had a nourishing meal in months. I guessed his height as 6 feet and his weight at about 140.

I introduced myself and explained that I was a surgeon and that Dr. Danielson thought I should consult on the case. He nodded his head. I asked him a few questions about his illness and got the same story Lennox had given me. He hadn't been eating much, he explained, because he hadn't been able to find steady work. It was when he had cut back on his eating that the stomach pains began. He also told me he smoked two or three packs of cigarettes every day.

I examined him, concentrating on his abdomen. I had noticed as we talked that his abdominal muscles barely moved when he breathed; he was moving air almost entirely with his chest, a sign of abdominal pain.

As soon as I put my hand on his abdomen, he squirmed. "Don't push on my belly, Doc," he said, "it hurts like hell."

"Don't worry," I said, "I'll be very gentle. I just want to see where it hurts the most."

The entire abdomen was tender, but the most sensitive area of all was in the midline just below the breast bone. I asked him if it hurt more to lie still or move around and he said, "To move around." Abdominal pain on motion suggests irritation of the lining of the abdomen, as in peritonitis from a ruptured ulcer or appendix. Patients with the severe pain of kidney stones usually prefer to pace around the room.

I finished my examination, excused myself, and met Lennox in the X-ray viewing room. There were three films on the view box; one of the chest, one of the abdomen with the patient standing and one of the abdomen with him lying down.

"What do you think, Bill?" Lennox asked.

"I'll guess what I'll bet you're guessing. I think he's got a perforated ulcer."

"Agreed," Lennox said, "but I don't see any free air in the abdomen." When a stomach or duodenal ulcer breaks open it not only causes exquisite pain but, usually, air in the stomach leaks out and collects underneath the right side of the diaphragm, the broad muscle sheet that separates the chest from the abdomen.

I studied the films. "I don't see any air either," I said, "but that's the case in about ten percent of perforated ulcers. (When I'm called as a consultant, I like to drop any little nuggets of information I've recently read or still remember from my student or resident days.) I suppose we could squirt some air down a Levin tube into his stomach, get more X-rays, and see if any air shows up outside his stomach, but personally I think his history is so good that I don't think we ought to waste any more time, I think we ought to operate right away. He probably perforated at four this afternoon which is almost nine hours ago, and the incidence of complications from a perforated ulcer start to climb rapidly after four hours. (A second nugget.) I'll bet you've had an amylase done?"

"Right. It's normal." A marked elevation of the

blood amylase, a digestive enzyme produced by the pancreas, would have suggested pancreatitis, inflammation of the pancreas, which is a disease best treated medically, not surgically. In fact, when a surgeon operates, thinking the patient has an inflamed gallbladder or a perforated ulcer, and finds instead an inflamed pancreas, the best thing he can do is to get out of the abdomen, and fast. Patients with acute pancreatitis can get very, very sick, and careful medical management is what they need. But it's the rare surgeon who doesn't, at least once in a great while, bump into a case of pancreatitis when he's expecting something else.

After I'd explained to Tommy what we thought the diagnosis was, and what we felt we should do to help him, he readily agreed to sign the operative permission slip. At 1:15 he was in the operating room, anesthetized, and we began. Usually I make generous incisions; there's an old adage that says "incisions heal from side to side, not end to end," but in patients with perforated ulcers I try to keep the incision short. For some unknown reason there's a high incidence of poor healing in perforated ulcer patients and the shorter the incision the less likely it is to break open, other things being equal. Besides, a surgeon doesn't need much room to repair a perforated ulcer. If he makes his incision properly and if the perforation is where it usually is, in the first portion of the duodenum just beyond the lower end of the stomach, he can close the hole, which is rarely more than half an inch in diameter, with one or two stitches. In Tommy's case everything went smoothly, we came right down on the ulcer and, "skin to skin," the repair took us just twenty minutes.

However, as I've mentioned, it had probably been at least nine hours since Tommy's ulcer had perforated and both Lennox and I were concerned that he was in for a stormy postoperative course. If you repair an ulcer within the first perforation, the chances are excellent that the patient will make a prompt recovery. But after those first four hours the possibility of complications, particularly abscess formation within the abdomen from collections of fluid, food and bacteria that have leaked out through the ulcer, increase. The overall reported mortality from a perforated ulcer is about five percent; but this includes cases operated on early, as most of them are. In cases where there have been relatively long delays, the incidence of complications must run to at least thirty percent and the mortality rate probably approaches five to ten percent.

Tommy had, on his side, his relative youth, but on the other hand he was obviously malnourished, which meant he probably didn't have much resistance to infection. Lennox and I talked about those things as we changed from our scrub suits into our street clothes. We put Tommy on antibiotics, hoping to stave off infection, but, other than that, there wasn't much we could do except manage him like any other postoperative perforated ulcer patient. We'd leave the Levin tube in his stomach for whatever time it took for the stomach and bowel to resume normal function and we'd feed him intravenously till we could get the tube out. By 2:30 we had explained the situation to Tommy's girl friend and I was home in bed.

For the first couple of postoperative days everything went as anticipated. Tommy's stomach and bowel didn't start to work immediately—sometimes within forty-eight hours of the repair of a perforated ulcer the patient can start drinking and eating—but we really hadn't expected Tommy to come around that quickly. We were delighted when, after four days, he started passing gas from his rectum, a sign his bowel was working again, and we were able to remove the Levin tube and start feeding him.

On the fifth day things began to sour. His temperature and white blood count, which had been just slightly elevated, started to "spike." His temperature would be normal in the morning, but by evening he'd be up to 102°. And his white blood count, normally 7-9000, rose from 12,000 to 22,000. We shifted him to a different antibiotic but we didn't expect it to help, and it didn't. Once an abscess starts to form, as we suspected was happening in this case, it has to be drained before the patient will get well. All the antibiotics in the world won't cure an established abscess.

Tommy, in the meanwhile, was becoming cantankerous. There's a phenomenon I've noticed dozens of times, a deterioration of the doctor-patient relationship, that occurs when patients develop complications. They want to get well, the doctor wants them to get well and yet they aren't getting well. Unconsciously, I suspect, the patient begins to blame the doctor because he isn't improving. The doctor, on the other hand, is angry at his own impotence. He's using all the weapons he has—in this case, antibiotics, intravenous fluids, even vitamins (which I give the patient only in desperation; I refer to them as ''witch doctor'' medicines)—and the patient doesn't get well. So the doctor begins to get angry, unconsciously, at the patient.

Tommy and I reached this stage on the eighth postoperative day. Earlier, on my twice-a-day visits, I'd been cheery and friendly and so had he. Now I was curt and impatient and he was surly. ''Goddammit, Doc,'' he said on the eighth day, ''what the hell is the matter? How come I still feel so lousy and run that temperature every day? You promised me I'd be better after a week.'' I had made no such promise; what I had said was that if everything went smoothly he should be better in a week.

But everything hadn't gone smoothly. I was reasonably certain Tommy was developing an abscess somewhere, and I hoped it would be in his pelvis, where it would be easier to drain than if it were up under the diaphragm, another common location for postoperative abscesses. ''Tommy,'' I said, trying not to lose my temper. ''I think you're getting a collection of pus in your abdomen. I told you that was a possibility, particularly since I didn't get to operate on you till nine hours after your ulcer perforated.'' This is another weapon doctors use on their patients when things don't go well; they put at least some of the blame on the patient. It's not a very nice thing to do, but we get tempted and we succumb. Never, I might add, in cases where we're certain the patient isn't going to make it. I'd never say this, for example, to a patient who was late in coming to me with cancer and who was dying because the disease was now widespread. ''I'm going to get some X-rays today to see if we can see anything to help us locate the abscess. I'm also going to do another rectal examination.''

''Not again,'' he said, groaning.

''Yes,'' I said, ''again. If you get an abscess in your pelvis, I may be able to feel it and even drain it through your rectum. That's why I've been doing these rectal examinations every day for the last three days. I know they're uncomfortable, but they're necessary. Let's go.''

On this eighth day, unlike the previous three, I thought I could feel a mass, like a baseball, pushing down on Tommy's rectum. I wasn't yet certain he was getting a pelvic abscess, but it was beginning to seem more likely. I decided to get the X-rays to see if we could detect signs of an abscess elsewhere—sometimes a pocket of gas, or an unusual shadow, or some displaced bowel will suggest the location of an abscess—but I was hopeful that by the next day I could be sure Tommy had a pelvic abscess.

The X-rays didn't help but the next morning, when I did the rectal exam (much against Tommy's wishes), I was reasonably certain I could feel a pelvic abscess. ''Tommy,'' I said, ''I think I can feel a collection of pus in your pelvis, lying on your rectum. Have you had any new symptoms lately?''

''Yeah,'' he said, ''I've been having diarrhea and even after I move my bowels I feel as if I have to go again." Those symptoms are common with a pelvic abscess, and I explained as much to Tommy. The pressure of the pus on the rectum narrows the passage so that diarrhea occurs; and the weight of the pus causes the sensation of incomplete defecation. (I realize that this is rather sordid subject matter, but so are pelvic abscesses. So, in fact, is a lot of medical practice. It's the doctor who skips the "sordid" things, like rectal examinations, who endangers patients.)

"Tomorrow, if you agree, we'll take you to the operating room and I'll try to drain that abscess into your rectum. We'll put you to sleep first, of course."

"You damn well better put me to sleep," Tommy said. "Once that's done I'll be better, won't I?"

"You should be," I said. "Usually once the abscess is drained the fever drops and you get better quickly."

"OK," he said, "but this better be it. I want to get out of here. My health insurance is lousy and I'm running up a hell of a bill."

"Don't worry about that now, Tommy, one thing at a time."

On the tenth day I drained the abscess into the rectum. I was delighted to be able to do so, because I knew that the relief Tommy would get would be just like that experienced when a patient has a boil drained. With the pressure gone the patient almost immediately feels better.

That evening when I saw Tommy we were buddies again. He already felt better and his temperature had stayed at normal levels all day. We were both delighted. "When can I get out of here, Doc?" he asked.

"Not so fast, Tommy. You're still weak as a kitten. We've got to get you built up so you'll be able to manage at home."

"All right," he said, "but not for too long. Ruth's been working in a grocery store since I came in here and she's saved some money. We can get all we need to eat now. I want to get home. I can lie around there."

So three days later, though he was still weak, I let Tommy go. I gave him a prescription for some vitamins, just in case he went back to his old non-eating, heavy-smoking habits, and told him to come and see me in a week. I wanted to keep a close eye on him during his convalescence. "There won't be any charge for your postoperative office visits," I said, "so don't let that possibility keep you away. I want to see you." I wasn't certain Tommy would keep his appointments, but I didn't want money to be the reason he didn't.

To my surprise he showed up promptly for his first appointment. He was still weak and wondered if there was something wrong. I explained that after what he'd been through it would take at least six to eight weeks to get back to near normal. He had dropped from an admission weight of 142 to 128 while he was in the hospital. I was pleased to see that he was already up to 131. I told him to check back two weeks later.

When he did he was much stronger. He was, by nature, a strong person. His weight was up to 137 and he felt much better. His blood count was normal and he was anxious to get back to work. I warned him against it. He'd need at least another month before his wound was solidly healed.

Then he asked me a question I suspected he'd eventually ask. "Doc," he said, "what about that jerk, Dr. Blank, who told me to go home and come back the next day. Couldn't I sue that bastard? I figure if I had done what he said I'd be dead now."

"I agree, Tommy," I said, "if you'd done what he advised I don't think you'd have made it. It was touch and go as it was. If the bugs in that abscess had gotten into your bloodstream you'd have been lucky not to have died. But as to whether you can sue and win, I just don't know. I'm not a lawyer."

"You think I ought to see a lawyer?"

"That's up to you. If it were me, I'd see one. I tell you that as a friend, not as your doctor."

"That's good enough," Tommy said. I gave him an appointment to come back in a month and he left the office.

About two weeks later I received a letter from an attorney I'll call Mr. Anthony asking me to send him a copy of all my records on Tommy French. A similar letter had gone to the hospital, both accompanied by releases signed by Tommy authorizing us to send the information to the attorney. About a week later I received a call from Mr. Anthony.

"I'm calling about a patient of yours, Tommy French," he said. "You've seen his release, I'm sure, so I wonder if you'd be willing to talk with me about the case?"

"Sure," I said, "I'll try to clarify anything not in the record."

"Thanks," Mr. Anthony replied. "It seems to me that this Dr. Blank was negligent as hell in not examining Tommy right away and seeing to it that he was admitted to the hospital."

"I agree. I think negligence is too mild a word for him."

"The problem as I see it," Mr. Anthony continued, "is whether or not we can prove that Tommy suffered as a result of this man's negligence. After he'd seen Dr. Blank, he got back in his car and his girl friend drove him immediately to the hospital where Dr. Danielson and you gave him prompt, appropriate treatment. Do you think we can prove that the outcome would have been any better if Dr. Blank hadn't sent him home?"

I hadn't thought about it that way. I was convinced that Blank was negligent and so was Mr. Anthony; but had Blank's negligence caused Tommy any harm? Blank's idiotic advice had been wisely ignored, so he really hadn't delayed proper treatment.

"You have a point," I said. "I guess I really can't say that Tommy would have done any better if he'd skipped his visit to Blank. Does that mean Blank gets off?"

"I'm afraid so," Mr. Anthony replied. "If we can't show any damages to Tommy then there's nothing to sue for. Blank was negligent, but no one was hurt. There's no case."

"Frankly," I said, "I'm sorry to hear that. I'd have welcomed a chance to testify against that s.o.b."

"You could still bring a complaint to one of your medical boards, couldn't you?" Mr. Anthony asked.

"I suppose I could," I said, "but that would mean getting Tommy and his girl to spend their time putting in a complaint and testifying. I don't know if they'll do it when they can't collect."

"Maybe we'll get him later," Mr. Anthony said.

"Maybe," I answered, "but I doubt it. I know this guy's reputation. He tries to treat nothing but colds and minor aches and pains. I don't know how he ever got a license in the first place."

"We have the same problem in my profession," Mr. Anthony said.

"Sorry I couldn't help." I said.

When I saw Tommy a week later I discussed the legal aspects of the case with him. He already knew there was nothing he could do to collect damages.

"I'd like to help you out, Doc," he said, "I'm no fan of that Blank's. The trouble is that I've got a job starting next week—light work for the first month, so don't worry—and I hate to have to take the time off. I'm up to my ears in debt as it is. That hospital bill was out of sight. And you won't be getting paid much for a while either."

"No problem, Tommy," I said, "pay what you can when you can. We won't press you. And I understand about your reluctance to testify. I'd probably feel the same. Anyway, we can be glad everything went as well as it did."

"You know," Tommy said, "there was a time in that

hospital when I was ready to strangle you. All those goddamn rectals. Now I'm so glad to be well I've almost forgotten them."

"I'm sure you could tell I wasn't too crazy about you either," I said, "Here I was, busting my guts to get you better and you were snarling every time I came into the room. Well," I said, smiling, "It's over now and we're friends. But for heaven's sake take care of yourself. The stomach X-rays we got before I discharged you showed that the ulcer was healed, but a fairly high percentage come back if the patient isn't careful. Try to eat regularly and stay away from the black coffee and cigarettes. You remember when I discharged you I gave you that spiel on what causes ulcers? If you don't want more trouble, don't abuse your body."

"Don't worry, Doc," Tommy said as we parted, "I had the hell scared out of me this time. I'm going to be a clean liver from now on."

We said goodbye and I haven't seen Tommy since. About a year ago I met someone from Walnut Grove who knew Tommy and he told me that he and Ruth were married now and living in Arizona. Tommy had apparently modified his life style after his narrow escape. I was glad to hear it. He wouldn't have lived long if he had continued to abuse his body. As it turned out—thanks to a girl friend who knew enough to ignore a jackass of a doctor, to the help we could give him in this hospital and, mostly, to Tommy's youth and his body's tremendous ability to fight disease—Tommy, having learned his lesson young, should be able to look forward to a long, hopefully happy, life.

Tommy's case illustrates, only too clearly, how helpless we physicians are in preventing diseases that result from abuse of one's body. We can preach till we're hoarse about the need to eat a decent diet, to get regular Pap smears, to exercise regularly, to keep one's weight at a normal level, to avoid cigarettes, but if patients choose to ignore this advice, that is their privilege. All we can do is try to remedy the ravages these practices make on their bodies. We have an obligation to try to educate our patients, but we have neither the authority nor the time to police our patients and regulate their life styles. In fact, we physicians are often as guilty as our patients of abusing our bodies in senseless ways.

6

The Liver Is a
Remarkably Resilient Organ

When I saw Charlie Lorenz, in consultation in 1963, he was one of the sickest patients I'd ever seen, another victim of flagrant abuse of one's own body.

Charlie's skin and the whites (sclera) of his eyes were so yellow they were almost orange. When our laboratory technicians tried to measure the level of bile (bilirubin) in his blood, they couldn't get an exact reading; there was so much bilirubin that the level simply went off the scale. All they could tell us was that it was "more than 25 mgms. (milligrams) in every 100 c.c.s (cubic centimeters) of blood." Normal levels in our laboratory ran to a maximum of 0.8 mgms. per c.c. (Each lab, depending on the equipment it has, the solutions it uses, and the procedure it follows, may have different "normal" standards. Usually, however, they don't vary much from one laboratory to another.)

I'd been asked to see Charlie by another doctor on the staff who I'll call Ralph, a general practitioner. Ralph wanted my opinion on whether Charlie's jaundice might be due to a disease that could be cured by an operation, such as removal of a stone or a tumor blocking the bile ducts and causing bilirubin to back up into the blood stream.

I didn't think so. It was hard to get a clear history from Charlie—his liver was in such bad shape he was almost in a coma—but simply by examining him and looking at the results of all his liver chemistry tests it seemed to me that, whatever was damaging Charlie's liver so badly, it wasn't obstruction. The liver function tests affected by obstruction are usually not the same as those affected by other liver diseases. It seemed to me most likely that Charlie's liver cells had been damaged directly, either by a virus, by alcohol, or by both. The liver performs many functions for the body—it produces proteins, helps metabolize food and medicines, acts as a storage place for sugar, produces substances used in blood clotting—that there are literally dozens of liver function tests that can be run in the laboratory which will help determine what sort of disease is damaging the cells. Sometimes, however, even after all the tests have been done, the diagnosis remains obscure.

However, there were several reasons why I was reasonably certain that Charlie didn't have a surgically remediable disease. He had had gallbladder X-rays a couple of years earlier that had shown a normal gallbladder without stones; he hadn't had any attacks of pain of the type usually caused by stones when they block off the bile duct; and, probably of equal importance, I knew Charlie pretty well and I knew that he was a very, very heavy drinker. By that I mean that Charlie probably consumed about a quart of whiskey a day. I also knew that he didn't eat very well or regularly. People who get most of their calories from alcohol are, eventually, going to wind up with damaged livers. Until recently we believed that this happened because, when the heavy drinker used alcohol as his only energy source, fat would tend to deposit in his liver, damaging the liver cells. We still believe this is true, but in the last couple of years we've also learned that alcohol, in itself, taken in large quantities, is toxic to liver cells. So, even if you eat a decent diet, the chances are pretty good that if you drink heavily you'll eventually damage your liver.

The question now becomes: What does the phrase "heavy drinking" mean? There are several definitions. Among the facetious definitions, two of my favorite are, "an alcoholic [to use another term for heavy drinker] is anyone who drinks more than his doctor," and "an alcoholic is any s.o.b. you don't like who drinks as much as you do." There are literally dozens of serious definitions of what qualifies a person for the label "alcoholic." My personal belief, and this is shared by many if not most physicians, is that there are great differences among individuals where tolerance for alcohol is concerned. One person may be able to drink a quart of liquor a day for years, without showing any deleterious effects; another, who drinks a pint a day for a few years, will wind up first with a fatty liver and then, if he or she continues to drink, a liver that will shrivel up into a mass of scar tissue (that will have become "cirrhotic").

A bit of a digression from Charlie's immediate case, it's true, but it seemed to me appropriate since newspapers and magazines frequently publish questionnaires that are supposed to help people decide for themselves whether they are alcoholics; most of these are harmless, a few even do some good by forcing the reader to recognize that he or she has an alcohol "problem," but none that I've ever seen takes into consideration the differences in individual ability to metabolize alcohol, so that none can be called definitive.

With Charlie, however, a fatty liver caused by excess alcohol consumption seemed a good bet. Although he was only forty, he had been drinking, at best local estimates, that quart of alcohol a day for eight years, and—unless he had an extraordinary tolerance for alcohol—this couldn't help but damage his liver.

I told Ralph what I thought, and he agreed. "Just thought I'd cover all the possibilities," he said. "I wouldn't want to have treated him for a booze problem and find out at autopsy that he had a big stone stuck in his common duct."

"I agree with you that he may come to autopsy," I said. "His liver function tests were terrible when he came in five days ago, but they're even worse now. And according to your notes he's becoming progressively more lethargic."

"No question about it," Ralph said. "He's harder to rouse now than he was shortly after he came in. What you may not have known, because I'm not sure I wrote a note about it on the chart, was that he went into the D.T.s [delirium tremens, a condition in which a patient suffering from alcohol withdrawal hallucinates, often develops a high fever, and not infrequently dies] the morning after he came in. He was seeing pink elephants and slamming around the room so that I had to sedate him for awhile. His wife, Anne, told me he admits to a quart of whiskey a day, but she thinks that on top of that he's been drinking a dozen cans of beer. And he's been at it for eight years. God, what some people won't do to destroy themselves." (As a general rule, whenever I ask anyone how much they drink I tend, mentally, to double the figure they give me. People who drink are generally reluctant to admit precisely how much.)

"Did he ever try to get off the stuff?" I asked.

"Anne told me that he joined A.A. about five years ago and stayed dry for six months; the six greatest months of her married life, she said. Then he went to a stag party one night, started drinking, and she couldn't get him to quit again. Neither could his friends in A.A., though they tried."

"How have they been living? I wouldn't think Charlie could earn enough doing odd jobs to keep them going."

"He couldn't, but Anne's parents had been helping out. Now that their kids are old enough—one's twelve and one's ten—Anne's got a job. I think she clerks in one of the local stores."

"If he makes it through this episode even Charlie might give up the booze."

"Maybe," Ralph said, "but that's a mighty big 'if.' As long as you agree it's not a surgical problem I'm going to put him on steroids. We've got nothing to lose at this point and they might help." Steroids—specifically cortisone or one of its derivatives—sometimes help people with severe, acute liver disease. Cortisone can cause side effects, such as fluid retention and stomach ulcers, but in desperate situations—and Charlie's was certainly desperate—there was little to lose by adding cortisone to his treatment.

To everyone's delight, Charlie began to improve. His stupor decreased, he became alert enough to eat (Ralph had been sustaining him with intravenous fluids containing sugar and vitamins), and three weeks after I'd seen him his jaundice had all but disappeared. Ralph asked me to do a closed liver biopsy on him. The pathology report read, "Fatty change and lobular hepatitis, consistent with alcoholic hepatitis." In the detailed description of the tissue there were reports of regeneration and healthy-looking liver cells, which was consistent with Charlie's clinical recovery.

When he was almost ready to go home, about a month after admission, Ralph "read the riot act" to Charlie. He told him explicitly that he had been darned lucky to survive. He warned him in no uncertain terms that if he ever went off the wagon again, it almost certainly would mean his death. "The liver is a big, strong, resilient organ, Charlie," Ralph said, "but it can take only so much. This episode undoubtedly destroyed some of your liver cells; how many, I can't say. But you'd better protect what's left or you're going to be in serious trouble."

"Don't worry, Doc," Charlie said. "I'm off the stuff for life. I've talked it over with Anne. I know I haven't given her or the kids a decent life. I've got a job lined up starting in two weeks. If I work at it, and I'm going to, I can be making pretty good money in a year or so.

"And I've rejoined A.A. Two of the guys who tried to help me the time I went off were up to see me yesterday. They're going to make sure I stay straight.

"Doc, I know what it is now to be damn near dead. No more of that for me."

"I hope not, Charlie," Ralph said, "not only for your sake but for your family."

For the next three years Charlie stuck to his guns. He didn't drink at all, as far as anyone in town knew; in Litchfield, unless you're a very, very, secret drinker, everyone knows who drinks. He was doing so well in his job—he sold farm implements—that the company decided to send him on the road. Charlie had a great personality and they thought he could help their company as a traveling salesman more than if he stayed in Litchfield. I knew Charlie pretty well and I warned him when I heard about the promotion that he'd have to be very, very cautious or he might go back to drinking.

"No problem, Doc," he said. "All that's behind me. I go out hunting with my friends, and when they drink whiskey I drink iced tea. I've been doing it for three years and haven't slipped once. If I thought there was any danger, I'd pass up this promotion, even though it means a lot more money, and we can use it because the kids are getting near college age. I appreciate your warning, but don't worry. I know I can handle it."

"I hope so, Charlie," I said. "It's your decision and I don't want you to think I'm butting in, but I know how awfully sick you were when I saw you in the hospital and I'd hate to see you back there again."

For two more years Charlie stayed dry. He was earning a lot more money than he had while in Litchfield and he and Anne had built a new home in a subdivision on the edge of town. Then, about six months after his home was completed, I heard rumors Charlie was drinking again. I asked Ralph about it.

"I'm afraid so, Bill," he said. "Anne came in to see

me last week and she told me he now thinks he can drink 'socially'; you know, have a couple, and then quit. She wanted him to come and talk to me about it but he refused—said there wasn't any problem and wouldn't be—which makes me as nervous as hell. But I can't drag him down to my office. We'll just have to wait and see.''

Six months later, in April 1971, we saw. Anne called an ambulance on a Monday night. Charlie had been drinking steadily for three days and, after waking up from a nap, started acting like a crazy man. Charlie reentered the hospital. He had the D.T.s again and was even sicker than he had been in 1966. Ralph had to use physical restraints just to keep him from slamming against the wall and injuring himself. Ralph worked on him for three days—resorting to steroids early, this time—and finally Charlie came around. His liver function tests were almost as bad as they'd been on his previous admission. For some reason which we never could figure out, he wasn't quite as jaundiced as he had been previously, but now, instead of a big, fat liver which we could easily feel through his abdominal wall, the liver was apparently only slightly enlarged. We guessed that a lot of it had been replaced by scar tissue.

During that admission, Charlie came as close to dying of liver disease as anyone I've ever seen. For three weeks he was, to use a cliché, at death's door. At one point Ralph thought of sending him to the University of Minnesota hospital to see if they'd consider him a candidate for treatment using a pig's liver, a procedure in which the patient's blood is run through an anesthetized pig so that the pig's liver can remove the waste products that have accumulated in the patient's blood, waste products the liver ordinarily breaks down and excretes. However, at the suggestion of the University consultant, Ralph first increased the steroid dosage in an attempt to see if that might make a difference. If not, Ralph would transfer Charlie.

The increase in steroids did the trick. Slowly, Charlie began to improve. It was another six weeks before he was off all intravenous fluids, eating well, and down to a minimal dose of steroids. After eight weeks I did another liver biopsy. The report this time read, "Fatty liver with many areas in which all liver cells have been replaced by scar tissue. Compatible with severe alcoholic cirrhosis." Again, in the detailed report, the pathologist mentioned that there were still some clumps of healthy liver cells scattered among the fatty, scarred areas. Apparently, since his liver function tests were back to normal, there were still enough of these healthy cells to keep Charlie going.

This time Ralph didn't say much to Charlie. "I guess it's pointless," he told him. "I warned you last time and you ignored me. I'm not going to bother even talking to you about it any more, Charlie. It's your life, and if you want to go straight from here to the liquor store, you can end it. You decide."

"I don't blame you for giving up on me, Doc," Charlie said. "I guess everyone has except Anne and A.A. I won't make you any promises. I thought I could get away with social drinking, but obviously I can't. I have two drinks and I'll take twenty more. You may not believe me, but I'm off it for good."

"We'll see, Charlie," Ralph said. "We'll see."

Amazingly, he has. It's nine years now since that last admission and he has been constantly on the wagon. He gave up traveling, which initially reduced his income, but a year ago he bought out the owner of the business where he has been employed, so apparently he's doing well. I think he'll stay dry from now on.

The liver is an amazing organ. It carries out functions that are much more complex than those of the heart, or even the kidneys, and it has fantastic recuperative powers. You practically have to beat it with a stick to destroy it.

In patients who have sustained severe injuries to the

liver, in a car accident, for example, it is sometimes necessary to remove half or more of the liver. Assuming the patient recovers from the operation, the cells in the remaining portion of healthy liver will do all the work that the entire liver did previously.

The liver also differs from many other organs of the body in that it has the ability to regenerate—i.e., grow—new cells. If you destroy some liver cells, others will grow to replace them. This is not true, for example, of the brain. If you destroy brain cells, no new ones will form. Why the cells of one organ are capable of regenerating while others are not remains a mystery.

It is also unclear why some people develop liver disease when they drink excessive amounts of alcohol, while others do not. I'll add one bit of solid, depressing information to complement Charlie's story. Shakespeare knew that, in regard to libido and potency, excessive alcohol intake "increased desire but diminished performance" in the male. Recent studies have added a scientific explanation for this well-known fact.

Physicians who were doing research on testosterone, the male hormone which, in ways yet unclear, affects sexual potency, studied a group of men in their twenties. These volunteers first had the testosterone levels in their blood measured and then drank about seven ounces (about four average highballs) of alcohol a day for periods up to twenty-five days. After five days the researchers checked their blood testosterone levels and found that they had dropped between twenty-nine and fifty-five percent. Presumably, at least, this would explain the diminishing potency that often accompanies excessive alcohol intake.

It is also true that most people, as they got older, find that their ability to metabolize alcohol diminishes. It takes fewer drinks to get them intoxicated. And the "hangovers," those horrible hours of headache, nausea, irritability, depression, insomnia and lack of ability to concentrate that follow any period of intoxication, become progressively more debilitating and prolonged. John O'Hara, who quit drinking entirely when he was forty-nine, wrote in one of his letters, "No one, absolutely no one, who has passed forty can remain unaffected by two martinis." I agree with O'Hara.

And though it is true that there are marked individual variations in the ability to tolerate alcohol, I am also very skeptical when someone who I know drinks heavily tells me, "I've never had a hangover." More power to them, if it's true. Frankly, I think it's baloney.

A final note. Charlie became an alcoholic with severe liver damage at the relatively early age of forty. After a few years on the wagon—staying away from alcohol completely—he thought he could go back and become a "social" drinker. It didn't work. Recently (in 1978–79) some physicians who work with alcoholics have suggested that what Charlie tried is possible; the reformed alcoholic, after a reasonable time, can resume social drinking.

On the other hand, most physicians who work with alcoholics feel very strongly that, if this is possible, it is possible only in rare cases and that the danger that the patient will regress to his or her former alcoholic condition is so great that the risk should not be taken.

Based on my experience as a physician in a small town, where over the last twenty years I've had a chance to watch local alcoholics who have later tried to drink "moderately," I agree with the conservatives.

7

The Luck of the Irish

George Doherty moved to Litchfield in 1969, when he bought a small drive-in restaurant on the south edge of town. He, his wife, Betty, and one of their five sons ran the drive-in during the late spring and summer; for the rest of the year George was on the road most of the time selling men's clothing.

I knew George quite well, not only because I had done a hemorrhoidectomy on him in 1970 but because Tim, one of his five sons, was a classmate and good friend of my oldest daughter, Jody. George—as you might guess from his name—is an Irishman. He grew up in and around Boston and moved to Minnesota in the late 1940's.

George liked to play poker and on Wednesday night —men's night at the golf club—he'd almost invariably be in the back room smoking a cigar, having a few drinks and playing cards, after a round of golf.

On October 25, 1971, George came to the clinic complaining of pain in the chest. "I had some soreness in my left shoulder off and on for the last week," he said, "but it wasn't really bad. I thought it was a muscle strain. Then yesterday I began to have pain on the upper left side of my chest. It's not too bad, but it's steady. That's why I thought I'd better come in."

One of my partners, Dr. Michael Murphy, who has

since left Litchfield to practice elsewhere, saw George and ordered an electrocardiogram. The electrocardiogram, commonly called an E.K.G., showed definite evidence of heart damage. George's pain was due to what is called a "heart attack." One of the arteries that supply blood to George's heart had become blocked, damaging the heart muscle. Michael immediately admitted George to the coronary care unit at the hospital and started him on the standard treatment for heart attacks; basically, oxygen, sedation, rest and continuous monitoring of the heart by electrocardiogram, so that if any disturbances of rhythm occur, the appropriate drugs can be given.

The "appropriate drugs" include such things as digitalis, quinidine, levophed, atropine, lidocaine and anticoagulants (blood thinners) such as heparin or coumadin. Which of these many drugs are used depends on the size and location of the damaged muscle, the patient's blood pressure and specific changes in heart rhythm that may occur. In any case different cardiologists may select different drugs to use, always taking into account the patient's size and the possibility that he may either be allergic or extremely sensitive to the drug. Drug choice and dosages must be wisely chosen and carefully monitored.

Otherwise, the treatment of a heart attack is fairly routine. The patient is sedated, so he will not be apprehensive. He is given a pain killer (usually morphine) to relieve the pain that usually occurs in the chest, shoulders, jaw and/or arm. Oxygen is administered, usually through tubes that fit comfortably into the nose, so that his blood will be as saturated with oxygen as possible, particularly the blood which reaches his heart muscle.

George's blood pressure on admission was 180/110. He'd known he had high blood pressure but, like so many patients with hypertension, he hadn't taken his medication regularly. "I take it whenever I think I need it," he said at the time. That is a story every doctor hears frequently; though, since hypertension produces no symptoms, how a patient can tell when he or she *needs* the medicine remains a mystery.

George's attack, though it caused a moderate amount of damage to his heart muscle, didn't cause any rhythm disturbances. He made an uneventful recovery and was discharged from the hospital on November 13, twenty days after his admission. Michael had put him on a diet—he was fifty-one years old then and about twenty pounds overweight—and had emphasized the need to stay on his antihypertensive medicines no matter how well he felt. George convalesced at home for three weeks, gradually increasing his activity, and then went back on the road.

On George's first day home from the hospital, while he was supposed to be on limited activity, his wife heard strange noises down in the basement. She went down to see what was causing them and found George jogging in place, soaking wet with sweat. "George," she shouted, "stop that. You're supposed to be recuperating, not running like a madman."

"I know, I know," he said, stopping to towel himself off. "It's just that I'm damned if I'm going to live my life as a cripple. I'd rather go quickly than hang around, barely existing." But Betty insisted and he finally quit. He had already proved that he could go all out, and that was all he really wanted.

I tell this story just to demonstrate the sort of guy George is—a "type A" in medical classification—a person who is time-conscious, driving, always trying to do more than there is time to do. He loves his work—running around the midwest, chatting with the store owners, selling men's clothing for the manufacturers he represents. It's a hectic life, but it suits him. He'd rather die than give it up.

Incidentally, I'm also a type A, as are virtually all surgeons. Type B, the only other "type," are the ones who live by the philosophy that there's never any need to rush, things will get done eventually and there's no sense knocking yourself out to do them. As my mother often says, "Come day, go day, God send Sunday." I've never really understood what that meant, but I suspect it's an old Irish saying that suggests hurrying is pointless; a day of rest is coming whatever you do.

Most doctors are, by nature and necessity, type A. Only pathologists, dermatologists and, to a lesser extent, radiologists, are often type B. They're the only doctors who can usually take their time about arriving at diagnoses and aren't under pressure to see patients promptly and treat them immediately so that they don't develop complications or, possibly, die. They have time to consult with confreres and share responsibilities. That takes a lot of pressure off.

You might think that doctors who do research would be type B, since theoretically they aren't under any pressure to produce results. But that isn't so. Most doctors engaged in research are extreme type A's. They want to be *first*—first to publish a breakthrough in medical research. They're looking for fame, often at the sacrifice of large incomes; and it's the person or team who accomplishes the job first that becomes famous. I'd suspect that only a rare reader knows who did the second or third successful heart transplant, but virtually everyone knows Christiaan Barnard did the first. And, to get out of the medical field, it's the rare individual who knows the name of the second person to fly the Atlantic solo. Yet virtually everyone has heard of Charles Lindbergh. Silly? Certainly. But a fact, nevertheless.

So you find that research doctors are almost invariably type A—the successful ones, certainly—and George, in his line, is a type A. Type A's, all other things being equal, are ten times as likely to develop heart disease as are type B's. This has been demonstrated, statistically, in countless studies by psychologists and physicians. The explanation suggested for the predeliction of type A's to develop heart disease is usually the stress they are under. No one knows with certainty that that's the accurate explanation, but it seems a reasonable one.

Now, back to George.

George continued to have occasional episodes of pain in his shoulder, a not uncommon occurrence in patients who have had heart attacks, but generally he felt well until April 26, 1972, about six months after his first attack. On that date the pain in his shoulder suddenly became very severe. He called Michael, who had him go directly to the hospital where he was admitted to the coronary care unit for observation. The electrocardiogram taken as soon as he was admitted showed that George had had another heart attack. (Second attacks most frequently occur less than a year after a first. No one knows why this is so.)

This time, things did not go well at all. Almost as soon as he was admitted to the hospital, George's heart stopped and had to be shocked before it would resume beating. He developed bizarre rhythm changes, a certain sign that there is damage to the nerve conduction system in the heart. Then his blood pressure dropped to shock levels and he went into heart failure; i.e., his heart was pumping so inefficiently that it couldn't keep the blood from backing up into the lungs. Dr. Murphy is an excellent internist, fortunately, and he managed George's case with great skill. He used a wide variety of drugs to support George's failing heart and manipulated the rhythm-controlling drugs like a juggler to try to keep George's heartbeat regular.

I'd drop in to see George almost every day, though sometimes he was so sick I didn't dare disturb him. When I asked Michael what George's chances were, he said, "Slim, at best. He's had a massive coronary, and any time a patient with a coronary goes into shock and heart failure the chances of recovering aren't very good."

George, however, on the occasions when I spoke with him, seemed very philosophical.

"Hell, Bill," he said, "we Irish are tough. I'll get through this thing all right."

"Sure you will, George," I said, but I didn't really believe what I was saying.

However, after the end of his second week in the hospital George did start to get better. The episodes of bizarre rhythm became short and infrequent and it was possible to discontinue the drugs that had been used to keep his blood pressure up. Michael kept him on digitalis—a drug that strengthens the heartbeat—but other than that he was off all medicines by the end of the third week. He was also out of bed and walking around. He was no longer in heart failure.

Five weeks after he was hospitalized he went home. I met him in the hospital corridor just as his wife Betty arrived. "What did I tell you, Doc," he said, "it's tough to kill an Irishman."

"I guess you're right, George," I said, "but for heaven's sake don't scare us again, will you? These attacks seem to be tougher on us than they are on you."

"Don't worry," he said, "I'm through with this nonsense."

Six weeks later he was back at the drive-in, cooking fried chicken, pronto pups, hamburgers and all the other things he sold. I chatted with him whenever I'd stop to buy a bucket of fried chicken to take home. He was feeling fine.

A couple of months later Michael referred him to a bigger medical center so that he could have an angiogram done. An angiogram is a procedure in which dye is injected into the coronary arteries, the arteries to the heart, to see if there is a localized obstruction to one or more of the blood vessels, in which case a coronary bypass operation can sometimes be useful in increasing the blood supply to the heart. George's angiogram showed no suitable arteries for a bypass. "Hopeless situation" was the verdict.

That was six and a half years ago. George sold the drive-in in 1976—he was tired of running two businesses—and in the summer of 1978 he and Betty moved to Shakopee, a suburb of Minneapolis. Most of their sons were living around Minneapolis and they wanted to be near their family.

George still travels, however, and last night (December 16, 1978) Joan and I met Don and Junice Larson out at the Litchfield Golf Club. Don owns Viren-Johnson's, a men's clothing store in Litchfield. "Have you seen George Doherty lately?" I asked Don.

"Saw him just two weeks ago," Don said, "and he looks the best he's looked since I've known him, and that's over thirty years. Told me he feels fine too. I think the best thing that could have happened to him was getting rid of that damn drive-in."

Even if we assume that Don's description is a bit of an exaggeration—it's hard to imagine anyone looking better thirty years after you've met him—it's apparent that George is doing very well.

In April 1972 we doctors thought it unlikely that George would live a week. Yet here he is, eight years later, still driving around the midwest, selling men's clothing, and feeling great. Which only proves again that the heart is a very strong organ; and that we doctors aren't very good fortune tellers.

8

More Proof That Doctors, Certainly the Author, Are Fallible

Sometimes patients die, or narrowly escape death, because of a physician's error in judgment. (One of my mentors, when I was a surgical resident, would invariably say, when we referred to an "error in judgment," "Don't give me that 'error in judgment' nonsense; just use 'mistake.'")

He was semantically correct, of course. Still, I think "error in judgment" is an acceptable phrase. When I operate on a patient I often have to decide between two or three modes of treatment, all of which are acceptable. After considering all the alternatives, sometimes I must make my choice in a very few minutes and proceed accordingly. If things don't go well for the patient, then both she and I may be in trouble; but have I really made a mistake, in the ordinary sense of the word? I'd say "no." I made what seemed the proper choice at that time, but it didn't work well. Maybe one of the other alternatives would have been better, but of that I can't be certain. Given the choice again—which never happens, at least in the case of a specific patient—I'd have chosen a different alternative, because the one I chose didn't work satisfactorily. "Error in judgment" seems to me more benign, more forgiving, than that harsh word "mistake." I think there are times when we're entitled to use it after something has gone wrong.

Mary Brennan is a case in point. Mary came to my office one afternoon complaining that she was "all tired out." At least ninety percent of the time when patients come in complaining that they are "all tired out," their problem is a psychological one—trouble with their family, their partner, or their job. During the last two winters Litchfield was almost solid with people who were "all tired out." We had two winters (1977–78 and 1978–79), during each of which we went for over sixty consecutive days without ever having the temperature rise above freezing, and most of those days started with temperatures in the range of 10-30° below zero. In February 1979 I even told Cecil Leitch, the physician for most of our family, that I was beginning to think I must be anemic, I was dragging around so. "Nonsense," he said. "You've got cabin fever just like the rest of us." I had my hemoglobin checked anyway. It was perfectly normal.

Back to Mary Brennan. My initial reaction when I heard her complaint was that she was just over-tired; at thirty-five Mary had six children all under ten. But one look at her made me wonder if there wasn't more to it than that. Her skin was extremely pale and even the blood vessels of her eyelids seemed unusually blanched. Even before I talked to her and examined her I asked one of our technicians to check her hemoglobin level, an approximate measure of her blood volume. Normal, in women, is about 14 grams per 100 cubic centimeters; Mary's blood level was 9.5.

No woman would make a better candidate for an ulcer than Mary. She had been born and brought up in St. Paul, the only child of a wealthy stockbroker and his wife. She was used to a comfortable home and had never had to worry about money. She was an attractive redhead and she always had the best of clothes, a car as a high-school graduation present from her parents, and was disappointed when she got grades lower than an A. I had learned all this about her when I had been called once to see her when she was sick with a migraine. Migraine headaches—and ulcers—are both relatively common in compulsive people, and Mary was nothing if not compulsive.

She had gone to Macalester College, a small but excellent school in St. Paul, partly, I suspected, because she was an only child and was as reluctant to leave her parents as they were to let her go. It was while she was at Macalester that she met Ray, who was studying agriculture at the University of Minnesota. They had fallen in love and had been married after Ray graduated. Mary had left Macalester at the end of her junior year and it had always bothered her that she hadn't gotten her degree.

Ray was a big good-natured fellow who was perfectly content farming the 240-acre farm west of Litchfield that he was buying from his father. For Mary the transition from an easygoing life in St. Paul to the perpetually busy life of a farmer's wife was, at first, challenging and enjoyable. But as she had child after child after child, the strain began to show. No young farmer earns a great deal and it was difficult for Mary to keep her children as well-dressed and neat as she had always been. Mary's family helped the young couple, but Ray was an independent sort and he didn't want an inappropriate amount of help; he didn't want anyone to think he was dependent on his wife's family. All this put Mary under great stress and I had often wondered if the stress might take a physical toll.

As I asked her questions it became increasingly clear that she was probably bleeding from a duodenal ulcer. She had been having stomach pain beginning about two hours after each meal for three weeks; the pain went away if she drank some milk or ate some food. She hadn't had any vomiting but for the last week she had noticed that her stools were very dark.

"Like tar?" I asked.

"Almost that black," she answered.

Dark, tarry stools are almost a certain sign of blood in the stool. We confirmed this when we did a test for blood in a stool specimen after I'd admitted her to the hospital, which I promptly did. I passed a Levin tube into her stomach and aspirated blood. She was presumably bleeding from her stomach or duodenum. I started her on an ulcer diet and the next morning we took X-rays of her stomach which showed a moderately large duodenal ulcer. (Duodenal ulcers are relatively rare in women; they are about ten times more common in men. But when they occur in women they are apt to be severe.)

Without going into detail, let me explain that there are two acceptable nonsurgical methods of treating a bleeding duodenal ulcer. One way is to sedate the patient, give her milk, antacids and, sometimes, medicines to reduce acid production. If the patient isn't vomiting, this is often the treatment the doctor will try first; patients dislike the discomfort of having a Levin tube running through their nose into the stomach.

Which is, essentially, the second nonsurgical method of treating a bleeding ulcer. We pass the Levin tube into the stomach and attach it to a suction machine to keep the stomach collapsed and acid-free. The objective of each method of treatment is to wait and see if the ulcer will stop bleeding.

First I tried feeding Mary milk and antacids and it quickly became obvious that wasn't going to work. The night of her first day in the hospital she started vomiting the milk, the antacids and blood. Her blood pressure dropped from 130/86 to 100/70 and her pulse went up from 86/minute to 110/minute, both signs that her blood level was dropping. I had already given her two pints of blood. Now I rechecked her hemoglobin and it was down to 8.0. Obviously, she was bleeding faster than we were replacing her blood. I decided to shift immediately to constant Levin tube suction to see if that would work.

At first the returns from the Levin tube were persistently bloody but, during that second night in the hospital, they became less so; more like old coffee grounds mixed with green bile and yellow gastric juices. In the meantime I had given her three more pints of blood—a total of five pints—and her hemoglobin level was up to 11.5 grams. Her pulse was down to 84 and her blood pressure was normal.

When I spoke to Ray, I told him I was pleased. I had talked with him several times during the three days Mary was in the hospital, explaining why we were managing her case as we were. By the third day he knew an awful lot about the anatomy and physiology of the stomach; possibly more than he wanted to know. (When patients have a serious disease, for which there are alternative methods of management, I try to be certain that both patient and family understand what I'm doing and why. Following that policy there are rarely any recriminations if, finally, I have to resort to what might be called radical measures.)

As it was, on this third hospital day, I told Ray and Mary, "I'm going to leave the Levin tube down for one more day. Then, if the bleeding doesn't recur, I'll take it out and we'll go back to the milk-antacid routine. Gradually we'll get you back to solid food.

"Remember," I added, "everything I've told you is subject to change if you begin to bleed again."

On day four there was still no blood coming back the Levin tube. Mary's blood level had stabilized at 11.0 gms. and she was smiling when I came into the room. "I get the tube out now, don't I, Dr. Nolen? I'm not bleeding, am I?"

"No, you're not," I said, "and, yes, I'll ask one of

the nurses to take out the tube." (It's not that I'm above removing a Levin tube, it's just that I invariably spill fluid on the bedclothes when I remove it. The nurses do the job more neatly than I do.)

During days five and six Mary continued to improve. I reduced her sedation, she was out of bed, she even went down to the lobby during visiting hours to see her children. On the seventh day I started her on soft food and she asked me how soon she could go home.

"Another day or two," I said, "providing everything goes well." I think my practice of always adding to promises phrases such as "providing everything goes well" is one many doctors use. It's sort of a throwback to the witch-doctor days. We're afraid if we don't equivocate, if we promise too much, something disastrous will happen.

In Mary's case something nearly disastrous did happen. The night of the seventh day, about 1:00 A.M., the nurse on Mary's floor called me. "Dr. Nolen," she said, "I thought I'd better phone right away. Mrs. Brennan's blood pressure was 126/86 at 10:00 P.M., and now it's down to 96/60. And her pulse has gone from 84 to 120. She hasn't vomited but she feels as if she might."

"Start an I.V. right away," I said, "just run in some 5% D/W [sugar in water] but make sure the lab has got at least three pints of blood crossmatched. Get someone over to check her hemoglobin and have a Levin tube ready." I got dressed and went directly to the hospital.

When I walked into Mary's room she came immediately to the point. "Do you think I've started bleeding again, Dr. Nolen?" she asked.

"I'm afraid so, Mary," I said. "We'll know for certain in a minute. I'm going to put that tube back down."

"Do you have to?" she asked. "I hate that thing."

"I know you do, Mary," I said, "but we've got to find out what's going on. The tube may be a big help to you. It was once, you remember."

When I passed the tube and aspirated the stomach contents, it was almost pure blood. By then the lab technician had a report on the hemoglobin; down from 11.5 to 9.0.

"No question, Mary," I said, "that damn ulcer is bleeding again. We're back to square one."

"What next?" she asked.

"Well," I said, "I'm going to give you a couple of more pints of blood and see if the Levin tube gets you to stop bleeding. If it doesn't, we may have to operate. You remember I told you at the very beginning that we might eventually have to take out part of your stomach if the ulcer didn't heal."

"But I'm so young," she said. "And I'm scared of the surgery."

"For the moment don't think about it," I said, "let's see what happens. I'm going to have the nurse give you a shot so you can get some sleep. You and Ray and I will talk later in the morning."

There are a lot of rules doctors try to go by when they're managing patients with bleeding ulcers. Some automatically operate if the patient doesn't stop bleeding in forty-eight hours. Others make it a rule to operate if they have to give more than six pints of blood. Most of us will operate more quickly on large ulcers, particularly if they're in the stomach rather than the duodenum. These almost invariably bleed heavily and, besides, it's relatively easier to remove a portion of a stomach containing a stomach ulcer than to do the proper removal of the lower part of the stomach and first part of the duodenum that duodenal ulcer bleeding requires. At one time or another—because of the age of the patient, the size of the ulcer, the patient's general physical condition, a shortage of blood of the proper type—most surgeons have broken one or all of these rules.

There is, however, one that is almost never broken. If a patient comes into the hospital bleeding from an ulcer, stops after medical treatment, and bleeding recurs while still on medical treatment a surgeon will—and should, barring very critical contraindications such as severe heart disease—operate. If the patient is going to bleed under the optimum conditions that prevail in the hospital, then she will almost certainly bleed again unless you operate and remove the offending part of the stomach. (A note is in order here: Even if the ulcer is in the first part of the duodenum, an inch or so below the stomach, the critical area to remove is the lower half or ⅓ of the stomach where the hormone that stimulates acid production is secreted.)

According to all the rules, I should now have operated on Mary. She'd bled about nine pints of blood; she had re-bled while on medical management; her general health was excellent. But the next morning, when I came into her room where Ray was sitting with her, I could see the bleeding had stopped. All that was coming back in the tube was green bile and yellow gastric fluid. Her hemoglobin, after the three pints of blood we gave her during the night, was back to 11.5 grams. She was all smiles.

"No operation?" she asked.

"Damn," I said. "You've got me on the spot. You know I told you earlier that if you re-bled I'd have to operate. But you've stopped so quickly and look so good I just don't have the heart to operate.

"OK," I continued, "it's against my better judgment but we'll give you another chance. Three days on the tube, then we'll feed you. Don't scare me again."

"Don't worry, Dr. Nolen," she said. "I know I've stopped for good this time."

How I wish she had been correct. Instead, five days later, when she was back on the milk and antacid routine, at seven at night she vomited—and I mean vomited—huge amounts of blood and milk. I called Ray, told him what had happened, and said, "No more delays, Ray. Mary agrees. As soon as we have five pints of blood crossmatched, I'm going ahead. Tonight. The operating room staff is already setting up the room."

"I agree, Doc," Ray said. "Tell Mary I'll be right in."

An hour later, after I'd called one of my partners to assist me, we were in the O.R. with Mary on the table. "Nothing to worry about now, Mary. We'll take part of your stomach out so you won't bleed any more, but we'll leave you plenty more so you'll be able to eat well."

"I'm sorry I talked you out of operating a week ago," she said.

"Not your fault," I said, "I'm the doctor. It was my job to persuade you and I couldn't even persuade myself. I should know better than to break all the rules. Don't think about that now. Chuck is going to inject something into your vein to put you to sleep, and next thing you know you'll be back in the recovery room wide awake. You'll be a little bit uncomfortable, but we'll give you hypos when you need them."

"How about this tube?"

"You'll need it for two or three days after surgery, but you won't mind it. You'll see."

With that Chuck put her to sleep and we went to work. I opened her abdomen with a midline incision from her sternum to her navel. When we got to the ulcer we could see a big vessel pumping right in its crater. It was stuck to the pancreas, so I just sutured it shut and then removed the lower third of her stomach and cut the vagus nerves, the nerves that run from the brain down along the esophagus to the stomach and help stimulate acid secretions. There are about a dozen different kinds of operations for ulcer—which means, as is the case whenever you hear of more than one operation for a disease, that no single one works in every case—but this operation, called an antrectomy (the antrum is the lower third of the stomach) and vagotomy, has a high success rate with few complications. It seemed to me the proper operation for Mary.

It took almost two hours—I'm a fast surgeon, and have done a gastrectomy in one hour, but this was a tough one—and Mary's postoperative course was not as smooth as it might have been had I operated a week earlier. She developed a superficial wound infection, possibly because her resistance was lowered by all the days she had spent without really good nutrition, and I had to leave the Levin tube down five days instead of the usual two or three because her stomach and bowel wouldn't start working as quickly as is usually the case. It was a long two weeks before she was eating solid food, up walking the corridors and, gradually, getting her strength back.

I talked to her, as I do all my patients, on the day she left. I explained that she'd be tired for another month or two, that I wanted her to eat frequent small meals rather than two or three large ones since the half of her stomach that was left needed time to expand, and that she should come in and see me in three weeks just to keep me posted on her progress. I also told her to call if any question occurred to her.

"I've got one right now," she said. "I hope you won't mind answering it. I could have died from that last hemorrhage, couldn't I?"

"You could have died from the first one, Mary," I said, "but if you're asking was it more likely that that third hemorrhage could have been fatal, I have to say yes. By that time your nutrition was lousy, almost all the blood in your body was transfused blood, which is never as good as your own, and you'd had two episodes of shock—periods when your blood pressure fell drastically—which doesn't help your heart or kidneys. Fortunately you were young and strong. Otherwise, I'm not sure you'd have made it.

"On the other hand," I added, "if you weren't young

and strong I'd have probably operated sooner than I did."

"I certainly thank you for all you did, Dr. Nolen," Mary said, "but I guess I ought to thank the Lord too. Maybe He thought I ought to be around to raise those kids," she said, smiling.

"I think we can both thank the Lord, Mary," I said. "This case taught me something too. From now on I won't let my emotions cloud my judgment, as I did this time."

That, of course, has subsequently proven to be a lie but I *swear* I meant it when I said it.

Mary hasn't had a bit of trouble in the two years since we operated. I think when her kids start to irritate her—and as the father of six I know those times are frequent—she remembers how close she came to leaving them and her natural good spirits return.

Sometimes it takes a tight squeak to make us count our blessings.

9

If You Lose Perspective, Call for Help

When we moved to Litchfield, Annie Jamison was one of the first nurses I met. In 1960, before we had the I.C.U. (intensive care unit, which was added to our hospital in 1973), if I had a patient who was, as the saying goes, "rocky"—i.e., in an unstable condition postoperatively, either because she was awfully sick, or awfully debilitated when we started the operation, or because the operation had been a difficult one or something had gone wrong during the procedure—I'd call in a special nurse to take care of the patient till she was stable. This might mean just one eight-hour shift or it might require several days with "specials" on each shift. (In the 1980's "special" nurses are a dying breed. Patients who need close supervision are generally put in intensive care units, where the nurse-patient ratio is rarely greater than one to two. "Specials" are called in only for those patients who don't need but want full-time nursing care; mostly the very wealthy.)

One of my first patients—a patient who had a cardiac arrest during a supposedly "minor" operation, an appendectomy—fell into this category. This might be a suitable place to mention that, as spokesmen for the American College of Surgeons often say, "there's no such thing as 'minor surgery, only minor surgeons,' " a view with which I was once not in entire agreement but one which, with experience, I have begun to endorse almost wholeheartedly. The message behind the slogan is "don't try to perform any operation unless you have the training to do the much bigger one which may prove necessary."

This patient, whom I'll call Pete Ringer, was fifty-six and we'd known he had advanced valvular heart disease and was in borderline heart failure, but when you get appendicitis it doesn't matter what other diseases you have—the appendix has to come out. I'd operated on him reluctantly and the operation had gone smoothly but, as we were closing the wound, his heart stopped. I massaged it, reaching up under the diaphragm from within the abdomen and squeezing the heart between the diaphragm and the ribs. We managed to get it going again, finished closing his abdominal wound, and sent him to the recovery room. Then I went and spoke to his family. I told Mrs. Ringer that everything was under control at the moment, but that I thought we ought to have a special nurse for Pete, at least for the 3-to-11 and 11-to-7 shifts. We could decide the next morning whether we'd need specials any longer.

The nurse who came on for the 3-to-11 shift was Annie Jamison.

Annie is tall and slender. At sixty-six there were only a few strands of gray in her black hair. She could easily have passed for fifty. Now, twenty years later, she still looks and acts like a much younger woman. Amazingly, she has never worn glasses and, since I often see her pedaling her bike around town and she never has any accidents, I assume she can see well without them.

Annie had worked a regular shift at the hospital till she was sixty-five and had been forced to retire because of the mandatory age requirements. I told her what had happened to Pete during the operation, and explained that we were particularly wary he might develop cardiac complications, so that we'd want her to check his pulse and blood pressure frequently.

"Don't worry about Pete, Dr. Nolen," Annie said, "we've known each other a long time and I won't let anything happen to him."

You could almost see Pete, who had understandably been very apprehensive, relax when Annie came into the room. "I'm sure I'm in good hands, Dr. Nolen," Pete said. "I feel better already."

As it turned out, Pete recovered without any further complications and I'm sure, in part, it was due to Annie's ministrations. Pete *did* relax when Annie was around and that relaxation was good for him. There's enough stress caused by an operation, particularly one in which a complication develops, without adding to it by leaving the patient in the care of a nurse he doesn't like or trust. Annie was so calm and good-natured that it would take a real Scrooge not to get along with her.

Over the next several years Annie and I worked together on many cases. When I asked Ruby Anderson, our nursing supervisor, to get me a special—often a sudden request, the result of an emergency situation—I was always pleased when she got Annie. Even though Annie didn't come to any of the G.P.s at our clinic for her care—she has always been a patient of Greg Olson's—I saw a lot of her because, as the only doctor who did "big" surgery, I often requested specials for a day or two in the postoperative period. I learned that she had a wry sense of humor, which I enjoyed, that she rarely if ever got ruffled, that she'd never bother you over trivia (she had a lot of common sense and wasn't afraid to use it), but that she also wouldn't hesitate to ask you to see the patient when she suspected something dangerous had happened. On top of all that she had a rare and beautiful quality; she liked people and when she worked with them she treated them cheerfully and with compassion. Altogether, an excellent nurse. I was sorry when, in 1970 at the age of seventy-six, she decided to retire.

Annie, like most people, had her share of ailments. Mostly minor. In 1971, shortly after she had retired, she slipped on the ice and broke her wrist. It healed without complications after Greg put a cast on it.

In May 1972 she went to see Greg, complaining of a "tired-out" feeling. He checked her over and found she was anemic: her hemoglobin level was down to 10.2 when, ordinarily, it should be around 14 (grams of hemoglobin per hundred cubic centimeters of blood). Greg admitted Annie to the hospital and did the appropriate X-ray studies of the upper and lower gastrointestinal tract. The only abnormality the radiologist reported was a polypoid growth. A polyp is a spherical structure, like a golf ball, that grows from the inner lining of the intestine on a stalk; the stalk may be a couple of inches or perhaps, just a fraction of an inch in circumference. Since this polyp was too far from the anus to be removed through a proctoscope and since it looked like the type we call a "villous adenoma," which may contain cancer, we decided we'd better operate on Annie, remove the polyp and, if it had cancer in it, we would do whatever else was appropriate; possibly we'd remove the segment of intestine in which the polyp was located. Annie was in generally good health so, despite the fact that she was seventy-eight, we felt we could safely operate on her.

After opening the abdomen, I could feel the polyp in the lower intestine. I made an incision in the intestine and was able to remove the entire polyp with a surrounding margin of what appeared to be normal bowel. The pathologist examined it under the microscope, decided there was no cancer, and we closed the bowel and the abdominal wall. Annie made an uneventful recovery and was soon back home.

Greg saw Annie twice over the next year with what he

thought were attacks of gallbladder inflammation. X-rays of the gallbladder were inconclusive; it didn't function as well as the radiologist thought it should, but he couldn't see any stones. Both attacks subsided with only minimal medical treatment.

Then, in February 1974, almost two years after we'd removed the polyp, Annie again became anemic. Greg admitted her for X-rays of the bowel and this time the X-rays showed what appeared to be a cancer of the large intestine in an area known as the "hepatic (liver) flexure." This was several feet away from the place from which we had removed the polyp. Even though she was now eighty, Annie was still in good health and, since we knew that if we didn't operate on her, her bowel would soon become completely obstructed, we prepared her for surgery. On February 3, 1974, I opened her abdomen and we found a large cancer of the bowel. There was no evidence that it had spread to the liver but it did appear to have broken through the bowel into the fat of the mesentery—the tissue in which the blood vessels run to the bowel—and there were also some large glands in the mesentery which I suspected might contain tumor. The hepatic flexure lies very close to the duodenum (the first portion of the small intestine), and I had to peel it off this portion of the bowel. I managed to remove the tumor, along with a couple of inches of normal-appearing bowel on either end, and was able to sew the two ends of the bowel together, restoring continuity to the intestinal tract.

Annie, once again, made an uneventful recovery. As I mentioned earlier, it isn't unusual for the elderly to be confused and disoriented for a few days after a major operation, but Annie never had this problem. On the first postoperative day she recognized me, asked how things had gone and even wondered how soon I'd be able to remove the Levin tube from her stomach. As I've said, she's a remarkable woman.

Unfortunately the pathology report was not good.

The tumor had broken through the bowel wall into the fat and one of the lymph nodes had cancer in it. Once a cancer has spread beyond the organ in which it started the chances of achieving a cure decrease by about fifty percent.

In Annie's case, however, there was one positive factor that had to be figured into the statistics; her age. In an eighty-year-old patient cancer is apt to be far less aggressive than in a younger one. The forty-year-old woman who develops cancer of the colon, other things being equal (as they rarely are), will be in greater jeopardy than an eighty-year-old.

Greg and I discussed the question of whether or not to give Annie anticancer drugs in the hope that they'd kill any cancer cells we might have left behind and decided not to use them. Anticancer drugs aren't very effective against bowel cancer and we felt that Annie's slim chances of benefiting from them weren't great enough to warrant making her sick or causing the inconvenience of the trips to the doctor's office for blood tests and other necessary treatment.

Twice in 1974, Annie had what were apparently gallbladder attacks—abdominal pain and vomiting—but they always responded to conservative management. In January 1975, gallbladder X-rays showed good function and no stones were visible on the films. The attacks seemed typical of the sort patients with diseased gallbladders have, but in view of the normal X-rays the diagnosis of gallbladder disease could not be made with certainty.

Over the next three years Annie had no severe problems. She lived alone in her apartment, did her own cooking and house cleaning, and I'd occasionally see her shopping in downtown Litchfield. She has a daughter and several grandchildren who would visit her, or she them, every few days. Every time I saw her she was her usual cheerful self.

In April 1977 Annie noticed a lump on her right

cheek, about half an inch in circumference. She thought it might be a skin cancer. Greg agreed with her diagnosis, and he removed the lump under local anesthesia. It was a skin cancer. Skin cancers are very common, and as long as they're treated before they grow to huge proportions are rarely life threatening. The pathologist reported that Greg had removed the entire cancer along with a margin of normal skin. Annie didn't even stay overnight in the hospital for that operation. She came in in the morning, Greg removed the lump, and she went home immediately after this fifteen-minute operation.

In May 1978, when Annie was eighty-four, she had another attack of abdominal pain associated with some vomiting—much like previous attacks. This time, however, she became jaundiced. Greg admitted her to the hospital on May 10 and, among other blood tests, he had the lab check for bilirubin in the blood. Bilirubin is one of the breakdown products of the red blood cells which are continually being destroyed, as they grow old and are replaced by new blood cells manufactured in the bone marrow. Normally bilirubin passes through the liver, is mixed with other ingredients, and is excreted as bile into the intestine. When the bile can't get out, either because the liver cells are not working properly or because the ducts which lead from the liver to the bowel are blocked, bilirubin backs up into the bloodstream and causes the yellow discoloration known as jaundice. Usually it's first noticeable in the sclera, the white part of the eye, and then, as it gets worse, all the skin becomes yellow. The normal level of bilirubin in the blood is between 0.3 and 0.8 milligrams percent of blood. The bilirubin in Annie's blood was 9.1 milligrams percent.

Greg got other tests of liver function, all of which suggested that Annie's problem was not disease of the liver cells but, rather, obstruction of the ducts leading from her liver. The most common cause of bile duct obstruction is a gallstone or stones stuck in the bile duct, but Annie had had gallbladder X-rays just one year before which had shown a normal gallbladder. Greg was concerned, and so was I, that Annie's obstruction might be due to recurrent cancer blocking off the duct. After all, her bowel tumor had broken through into the fat and had spread to the gland only about two inches from her gallbladder.

The following day when I went in to Annie, she was sitting up in bed eating her breakfast.

"Sorry to bother you, Annie," I said.

"That's quite all right, Dr. Nolen," she answered, "I'm all through eating anyway. Who wants toast without any butter on it? Ugh!" Greg had put her on a fat-free diet, the usual practice for people with jaundice, since bile is important in the digestion of fat and if it isn't reaching the intestine, digestion of fats is impaired.

I sat down on a chair beside Annie's bed. "Tell me all about this business, will you, Annie?" I asked. "Tell me, for example, are you sure this jaundice hasn't been coming on gradually rather than starting with the pain in your abdomen?" The insidious onset of jaundice, without pain, would suggest a slowly obstructing cancer as the cause, rather than the sudden onset that occurs when a stone sticks in the duct.

Unfortunately, Annie's history wasn't much help. She admitted that her daughter had wondered if she hadn't been a little bit jaundiced a few days earlier, but Annie herself hadn't noticed it. When I'd finished talking with and examining Annie I still couldn't be certain what was going on. As I was leaving she did say, however, "One thing's certain, Dr. Nolen, I feel better today than I did yesterday."

"That's a good sign, Annie," I said. "I think we'll wait a few days and see how you do. It may be necessary to operate, you know. If you've got something blocking your bile duct and it doesn't go away, we're going to have to unblock you. But it's not an emergency. We'll check you and your blood for the next few days."

Later that morning the report on Annie's blood showed that the bile level had dropped from 9.3 to 5.8 and, as I said in my consultation note, "It is my feeling that in view of her age I would observe her and operate only if necessary. I suspect that, despite the negative X-ray, she may have had some sludge in her gallbladder." I was hoping Annie would get better spontaneously. I had no desire to reoperate, particularly in an area where I had previously done surgery and knew, from experience, there were likely to be all sorts of adhesions.

Unfortunately, Annie's lab reports got progressively worse. Perhaps the drop to 5.8 was a laboratory error. Our laboratory does excellent work but, even in the best of laboratories, errors occasionally occur. On the 17th her bilirubin was up to 10.3, on the 19th it was 13.4 and on May 20th it was 22.5. Not only was her jaundice increasing but Annie was beginning to slip. Her appetite was gone—not unusual in jaundiced patients—and she was rapidly getting weaker. Another day of deterioration and we wouldn't be able, as one of my professors used to say, "to cut her hair without killing her."

But now I'd reached a point where my objectivity was gone. Was it reasonable to operate on an eighty-four-year-old woman who, based on X-rays taken a year earlier, supposedly had a normal gallbladder, when she seemed to be rapidly approaching a painless death? Was I being falsely heroic in proposing to open the abdomen of this woman to try and help her? Was the evidence so certain she had a fatal condition that I ought to let her die in peace? I was too close to the case to be objective any longer. So was Greg. We decided to ask another doctor, Cecil Leitch, who hadn't till now known anything of the patient, to give us his opinion.

Cecil has always been a level-headed person. He was glad to consult. He talked to Annie, examined her, looked over her chart, listened to us describe her course, and then said, "No question, Bill, as I'm sure you already know. You ought to have a look, and right away. Maybe you won't be able to help her but you'd feel terrible if she died and at autopsy you found you could have saved her. She's tough. She can stand the operation. And she's been living a full life up till now. She deserves a chance to keep going.

"If she were senile or bedridden I might feel differently, but for this patient I think an operation is the right answer."

I thanked Cec for his consultation and then Greg and I talked the situation over with Annie's daughter, Jean. "Your mother is not a good surgical risk," I said. "At her age, few people are. But the way things are going she's just going to go progressively downhill. I don't know what's causing the jaundice. It might be a stone, it might be cancer. We can't get any helpful X-rays because when the bile accumulates in the blood, the dye we use to get gallbladder X-rays won't pass through the liver either. All we can do is operate and hope we find something that we can do to help her. It's my opinion—and that of Dr. Leitch, who we asked to see your mother just to give us another opinion—that we'd better operate now. Another day and she may be too weak to take it."

"Have you asked my mother about this?" Jean asked.

"I have," I answered, "and what do you think she said?"

"I know," Jean said, smiling. " 'It's up to you, Dr. Nolen.' "

"Right," I said, smiling too.

"Then go ahead," Jean answered. "And don't worry, Dr. Nolen—or you, Dr. Olson—I know you're doing what you think is best. If it doesn't work out, we'll understand." People usually do.

That morning we explored Annie's abdomen. We found a gallbladder as big as an orange—about four times the normal size. I felt the duct and couldn't feel any stones. There were, as I had suspected there would be, thick adhesions all along the bile duct in the area where we'd operated before but I couldn't feel any hard lumps that would have suggested a recurrence of cancer.

"Greg," I said, "it will take at least two hours and probably a lot of blood loss to uncover that bile duct up where we can explore it. I don't think Annie could stand it. Since her gallbladder is so distended it's obvious that bile is getting at least that far. Maybe she's blocked off by a stone at the end of the duct; maybe by cancer, though I doubt it since I can't feel anything hard and there's certainly no tumor in her liver. What I think I'll do is bring a loop of her jejunum (the upper part of the small intestine) up and hook it to the gallbladder. Then, even if the stone or whatever it is down below that's blocking off her duct doesn't pass spontaneously into the bowel, bile can get from the gallbladder into the intestine. That shouldn't take more than a half hour and it ought to solve her problem. What do you think?" Surgeons always like to have their assistant agree with them; then, if things don't work out as satisfactorily as the surgeon hopes, he can always say (at least to himself), "Well, my assistant agreed we were doing the right thing." Greg agreed.

I lifted the intestine up, and had it attached to the gallbladder in about twenty minutes. To make the connection, we had to open both the intestine and the gallbladder so that the gallbladder could drain into the intestine. When we opened the gallbladder it contained some thick bile but no stones; still, a small stone, or some sludge, might have passed from the gallbladder into the bile duct blocking it off. The entire operation took just one hour and five minutes. Annie's blood pressure and pulse rate remained normal during the procedure. It couldn't have gone more smoothly.

After the operation we decided to keep Annie in the I.C.U. for a day or two. At eighty-four, even an operation that goes smoothly takes a toll on a patient and I wanted Annie to have close postoperative supervision. Greg and I explained to Jean and one of her sons what we'd found, what we did and why. I drew a picture of the operation, since I've learned that is one of the easiest ways to explain things to patients or their families. I also warned them, as I always do, that things can go wrong postoperatively—delayed hemorrhage, blood clots that go to the lung, wound infections—and that, though we didn't expect any such problems, Annie wouldn't be "out of the woods" for at least two or three days. Jean and her son understood.

As it turned out Annie sailed through the postoperative period. I pulled her Levin tube out on the second postoperative day and by the third postoperative day we felt safe in moving her out of the I.C.U. into a regular room. Her bilirubin dropped from 22.0 to 3.5 in the next week and when we discharged her, fifteen days after the operation, she didn't have a trace of jaundice. She felt fine except that, understandably, she got "a little tired if I walk around too much." She spent the first week out at her daughter's home but then returned to her own apartment.

It's now twenty-two months since her operation. I met her daughter downtown (as we say in Litchfield) last week and she told me that Annie, now almost eighty-seven, was as active and bright as ever. "She hasn't had a bit of trouble since the operation, Dr. Nolen," Jean said. "Thank the Lord you decided to operate."

I didn't say "Amen," but I felt like it.

10

Tougher Than a Boiled Owl

One morning as I was sitting in the doctor's dressing room waiting for a patient to be brought down from the third floor to have a hernia repair, I went over the record on Joe Duclos. Here, from his admission on August 30, 1978, is the history as written by his family doctor, one of my partners, Dan Johnson.

Present Complaint: Can't breathe.
Present Illness: On day of admission patient was chasing cows which were out in his pasture, which hadn't been grazed, and the weeds were about chest high. He finally got the cows rounded up and proceeded to go out and pound a number of steel fence posts into the hard ground. Within a few hours he became extremely dyspneic [short of breath], cyanotic [complexion became blue], and was seen first in the emergency room and then admitted to the hospital.

Joe was sixty-seven in August 1978 and he has had emphysema (overdistended, inefficient lungs) and asthma for many years. Still, he's a tough bird—"tougher than a boiled owl," to use a favorite phrase of my partner, Harold Wilmot—and his chronic lung disease hasn't stopped him from running his farm. He's still in business.

What is, to me, most interesting about Joe is that on August 14, 1973, I operated on Joe. About a week earlier he had come to the clinic to see Dan, complaining of a lump over his right collarbone. "I've had it about four months," Joe said. "Hasn't bothered me at all and I thought it was just a bruise, but over the last three to four weeks it's been growing fast. Thought I'd better have you take a look at it."

Dan examined him, then had me check it. The lump lay beneath the skin over the collarbone (clavicle), and it seemed to me to be fixed to the bone, i.e., I couldn't slide the lump around under the skin.

"I don't know for sure what that is, Joe," I said, "but one thing's certain—it doesn't belong there. I think we ought to get some X-rays of your shoulder and chest and then we ought to take it out. It may be just a blob of fat or a cyst, but it doesn't feel like either of those things to me. It's possible it's a tumor of some sort."

Joe agreed to come into the hospital, where X-rays of the shoulder and of his lungs were normal, except for the emphysema which showed up on X-ray as oversized lungs less dense than normal. We wanted to make certain that if this was a tumor, it hadn't invaded the bones of the shoulder or spread to the lungs. As far as we could tell, it hadn't.

Joe wasn't the best surgical risk, because of his chronic lung disease, but this mass—which was about the size of a plum, about three inches in diameter—was too big to take out under local anesthesia. We figured Joe could tolerate what we hoped would be a short operation under general anesthesia.

On the morning of August 14, 1973, with Joe asleep, I made a four-inch incision through the skin over the mass. Then, with Dan assisting me, I tried to separate all the muscles and fatty tissue from the mass so I could, hopefully, remove it in one piece. Unfortunately, its wall was thin and I could see what looked like mucus inside it. When I was trying to free the tumor from the clavicle, to which it was firmly stuck, I broke into it and mucus spilled out into the wound. I kept working and after twenty minutes I'd removed all I could see of the wall of this tumor, though I knew I'd left at least a small part of the wall stuck to the clavicle. I wasn't going to remove a portion of the clavicle—a procedure which would have converted this relatively minor operation into a major one—till I knew whether the tumor was benign or malignant. After tying off a few small blood vessels I closed the muscles over the clavicle, then sutured the fat and skin.

Unfortunately, the report showed that the tumor was a myxoma, an odd sort of semimalignant growth. The pathologist, in his report, said, "This tumor can be expected to be locally aggressive with recurrence if not completely excised." In other words, since I was certain I'd left tumor stuck on Joe's clavicle, we'd have to reoperate on him and put him through a major procedure—one which, because of his emphysema, would be very risky for Joe—or we could expect the tumor to recur rapidly, possibly to the point where it would invade some of the major blood vessels that run behind the clavicle to the arm. This would be disastrous for Joe.

Joe made an uneventful recovery. However, when the pathology report came back on the 17th, and I told Joe what the pathologist had said and explained that we really ought to do another more extensive operation, he refused.

"No thanks, Doc," he said. "I need this shoulder to work the farm and I'm not going to lose any part of it. As far as I'm concerned, that lump is gone and I expect it will stay gone. Let's not go looking for trouble."

Frankly, I wasn't anxious to reoperate on Joe. He

was, as I've already said, a very bad risk. I felt I'd fulfilled my obligation to Joe when I told him what the pathologist had written and explained what it meant. I didn't try to talk him into another procedure. Dan sent him home on the fourth postoperative day with instructions to come in for stitch removal the next week and, as is usual after surgical cases, to come back to the clinic and see me in six weeks so I could be certain the wound had properly healed.

Joe came in to the clinic six weeks after the operation and his wound was fine. "Joe," I said, "I think you'd better come back to see us in three months. We're anxious to see if this tumor recurs." At the time of his six-week check I could still feel a small lump under the skin and I wondered how fast it would grow.

Three months later, when Joe came in, the lump, instead of being bigger, was smaller. I called Dan into my office and he checked it too. "Joe," Dan said, "You seem to be a very lucky guy. We'll want to see you again in six months—and, of course, come in sooner if your emphysema and asthma get worse—but, for now at least, your tumor troubles seem to be over."

In January 1980, I asked Dan if he'd seen Joe recently. "Saw him two weeks ago," Dan said. "Chipper as ever."

"Any trace of that tumor?"

"None," Dan said. "Oh, there may be a little bit of thickening underneath the scar but nothing startling. There certainly hasn't been any regrowth since you operated on him."

"Some guys are lucky, aren't they?"

"They sure are," Dan said. "And frankly, we're lucky we didn't do any more to Joe than we did. Obviously, he didn't need it, and we might have killed him."

"No doubt about it," I agreed. "But I sure thought he was all done when he said no to that second procedure."

Now why didn't Joe Duclos' tumor recur as the pathologist predicted it would? I can only speculate.

First, perhaps I did get all the tumor out initially, though I certainly thought I was leaving some behind on the clavicle.

Second, we know that tumors do spontaneously regress. I'll write more about that later, when I discuss another case, but in Joe's case I only mention it as a possibility. We don't know what causes most kinds of cancer; equally, we don't know why, once in a while, one we've left behind just shrivels up and dies. But we do know it happens. (Not, let me emphasize, often enough so anyone should hope it will happen when there is surgical, drug, or X-ray treatment available to treat their cancer without too much distress and with a significant chance of cure. For example, we can probably cure, surgically, about seventy percent of all breast cancers and virtually one hundred percent of cancers of the uterine cervix when they're found early. Spontaneous regression takes place, as best we can estimate, about once in every hundred thousand cases. Obviously, orthodox therapy is to be preferred to waiting for something we don't understand to, hopefully, happen.)

Third, it might be that in Joe's case even though I left behind some small patches of tumor, I might have destroyed the blood supply to these patches while I was cutting down to and removing the mass. Even tumors need oxygen to survive, and if there isn't any oxygen-bearing blood going to the tumor, it will die. That's the third and final explanation I have to offer for Joe's continued tumor-free survival after what I'd ordinarily consider an inadequate operation for an odd tumor.

As Dan and I agreed when we talked about Joe, he is one lucky man.

11

"God Helps Those . . ."

The last time I saw Ed Sletten was in August 1979. It was a Friday afternoon and Joan and I were just about to tee off on the tenth hole at the golf club when Ed drove up in his cart. He had just finished playing the first nine holes and was heading for his home, which is only a few blocks from the course. He looked well and I asked him how he felt. "Still a little weak, Doc," he said, "but not too bad for an old duffer. I expect I'll be getting stronger soon."

I assured him he would, then said goodbye as he drove off toward his home. "There's one guy," I said to Joan, "who I never expected to see out on the golf course again. I'll tell you, he's one tough cookie."

I've known Ed casually since 1964, as well as most people get to know someone with whom they have no close association. It was in 1964 that Ed returned to Litchfield after retiring as president of a bank in Butte, Montana. I got a brief summary of Ed's career from his wife, Valborg, when I talked to her on January 2, 1979.

Ed was born in Willmar, Minnesota, a city of about 15,000, thirty-five miles west of Litchfield, on April 10, 1889. He started his banking career in Litchfield in 1910, when he was twenty-one. After moving first to Brainerd and then to Albert Lea, with progressively increasing responsibility (including the presidency of the Albert Lea bank) he became, in 1945, the president of the bank in Willmar, a position he held till the mandatory retirement age of sixty-five, which he reached in 1954. Twelve days after he had to retire as the president of the Willmar bank he accepted the job as president of the bank in Butte, Montana. He held this job for ten years till he was seventy-five, then returned to Litchfield, the city he apparently liked most. He bought a house near the golf club so he could drive his golf cart to the course when he wanted to play.

I didn't meet Ed professionally, i.e., in my role as a surgeon, till May 5, 1975, at which time Ed was eighty-six years old. I'd seen him out playing golf and I'd chatted with him at the clubhouse when he and his buddies had stopped in after a round, but I didn't know him well, certainly not as well as I've come to know him in the last four years.

Ed has, since his return to Litchfield, always had Harold, who I've mentioned before, as his doctor. (I'm going to digress here for a moment. It seems, in my experience, that patients tend to go to doctors who are about the same age as they are. The explanation seems to be that people relate best to their peers. Obviously, some go to a doctor looking for a father or mother figure to advise and console them. But, the elderly particularly, like to go to an older doctor because he or she can relate to their complaints. Harold's older patients —remember, Harold is eighty—are the most loyal of all those who come to the clinic. Often, if Harold is away on vacation or out with a minor illness, these older patients will refuse to see another doctor. They'd rather wait till "their" doctor is back.)

In late February 1975 Ed came to see Harold. He was complaining of "sciatica," a general term applied to pain in the lower back radiating down the back of the leg. Harold examined him, didn't find anything specific and treated him symptomatically with aspirin. In about a week Ed felt better.

Then in March he began to feel weak. Nothing specific, just a general tiredness. On the 21st of April he came in to see Harold again. "Harold," he said, "something must be wrong with me. I couldn't bowl worth a darn in March. Almost too weak to throw the bowling ball. And every now and then I'd have to hire someone to shovel my driveway. It was all I could do to shovel my walk." As Harold noted in his physical examination notes, Ed "seemed to have lost his usual pep." As you can see, at eighty-six Ed was still accustomed to going strong.

Harold checked Ed's blood level at the clinic and found his hemoglobin was down to 8 grams. Ed was anemic. Harold put Ed in the hospital and ordered some tests to see if he could find the cause. One of the first studies, a barium examination of the stomach, provided the answer. The radiologist's report was "primary neoplasm [tumor] of the stomach until proven otherwise." It looked awfully big on X-ray. The radiologist said it involved "the majority of the mid-body of the stomach."

Harold asked me to see Ed. I talked with him and examined him and couldn't find any evidence that the tumor had spread beyond the stomach, though only if we operated on him would we be relatively sure it hadn't spread to the liver or some of the glands near the stomach.

"Looks like you need an operation, Ed," I said. "The radiologist says you've got a tumor. Almost certainly it's a cancer and it's bleeding. If we don't get it out of there, you're going to need transfusions all the time and eventually it will kill you." When it comes to talking to patients about the need for cancer operations, I vary, of course, with the patient's personality, but generally I'm fairly forceful. It's not like a hernia or gallbladder disease when, if the patient chooses, he can live with his discomfort.

"You know I'm eighty-six, Doc, don't you?" Ed asked.

"Sure I do, Ed," I said, "but you're a tough eighty-six. I think you can take this operation without any trouble." Which was the truth. I never lie to a patient.

On May 8, 1975, we operated on Ed and found a large cancer in the middle of his stomach. As far as I could tell, as I looked around in his abdomen, although the cancer had broken through the stomach wall into the fat next to it, it hadn't spread to the liver, the lymph glands or any other organs. I was able to leave enough stomach above the tumor so that Ed would be able to eat small meals comfortably. Even if you have to take out most of the stomach, and I estimated that I took out seventy-five percent of Ed's, the remainder will gradually expand so that the patient can eat meals of almost the normal quantity without any difficulty.

I also noted, while I was operating, that Ed's gallbladder contained a few stones, but since he hadn't had any gallbladder trouble I decided to leave it alone. It would probably be enough of a job for an eighty-six-year-old man to recover from the major operation I'd just performed.

The decision on whether or not to remove a gallbladder that contains stones, when the stones are discovered incidentally during an operation being done for another reason, is a matter of judgment. If the operative incision is located, as it was in Ed's case, in a place where the gallbladder can be visualized with relative ease, and if the primary operation has gone smoothly, then the surgeon may elect to remove the gallbladder since it is known that a gallbladder which contains stones will probably, eventually, cause trouble. But Ed had lived eighty-six years without any apparent gallbladder difficulty; if he had been forty I'd probably have removed it.

The reason for "incidentally" removing a diseased gallbladder electively is, as we shall see, so that the surgeon won't have to operate on it later under less favorable circumstances. Removal of a gallbladder is never "simple," but when it isn't inflamed it is usually not a difficult operation under optimum circumstances. Since it is a dispensable organ—it is a sac attached to the under surface of the liver and serves as a storage place for bile. It contracts and squeezes the bile out into the common duct and down into the intestine, after the patient eats a meal, to help with digestion—like the appendix it is often removed just so it won't cause later trouble. (I am assuming, of course, that the gallbladder contains a stone or stones; otherwise its incidental removal would not be justified.)

Except for some mental confusion during the first three postoperative days—a very common occurrence in the elderly, probably due in part to finding themselves in unfamiliar surroundings—Ed sailed through the operation. I sent him home, eating, in good spirits, and with a normal blood level on May 19th, eleven days after his operation.

A little over a year later I removed a small skin cancer from Ed's left temple, an operation I performed in the outpatient department. At that time, more than a year after his operation, Ed was feeling fine. I'd often seen him riding back to his home from the golf club.

In October 1977, much to my dismay, Ed developed abdominal pain and jaundice. Harold admitted him to the hospital and we ordered blood studies which suggested that his jaundice was due to a blockage of the duct through which bile flows from the liver to the bowel. I knew that Ed had gallstones and that possibly one might have slipped into his bile duct; but it was also possible—even likely—that the block was due to a recurrence of his stomach cancer. When stomach cancer recurs it often blocks off the bile duct.

However, Ed's jaundice gradually got better, which

made a stone a better bet than cancer; jaundice due to cancer rarely gets better. In any case, Ed's symptoms subsided and we decided to let him go home, hoping that perhaps only a single stone had caused the trouble and that he might now be trouble-free as he had been for so many years.

Unfortunately, the remission didn't last long. In the middle of November 1977 Ed had another attack of pain and jaundice. Since he still seemed to be in generally good health I told him I thought we ought to operate. "It's possible that it's cancer, Ed, but I doubt it. I think that damn gallbladder of yours is acting up. I probably should have taken it out when I operated on your stomach, but since it hadn't bothered you in eighty-six years I hoped it never would."

"You're the doctor," Ed said. "If you and Harold say I need an operation I'll take your word for it. Let's get at it."

On November 28, 1977, with Ed now eighty-eight, I operated on him again. To my great delight there wasn't a trace of cancer in Ed's abdomen. The gallbladder, as I had known it would be, was filled with stones and sludge and I removed it. Then, since I was reasonably certain one or more of the stones had passed from the gallbladder into the common bile duct, a hollow, tubelike structure ordinarily about twice the circumference of a pencil, I opened the duct and, using special "stone forceps," removed bits and pieces of stone from the duct. Then I put a T-shaped tube into the duct, one short limb extending up toward the liver, the other down toward the bowel, and brought the long portion out through the abdominal wall. I injected dye into this tube, after suturing the duct around it, and we took X-rays. The X-rays showed that the dye passed freely up into the liver and down into the intestine; we had relieved Ed of his bile duct obstruction and now, we expected, he would be free of future problems with jaundice. He would certainly never have any more gallbladder problems, since his gallbladder was now gone.

Ed's postoperative course was, once again, complicated only by the fact that he became disoriented for the first few days following surgery. In fact, after twelve days, even though he would occasionally recognize his wife or Harold or me, he often didn't know us and, most of the time, was confused about where he was and what had been done to him. I decided, after talking the problem over with Valborg that, since Ed had made an otherwise successful recovery, I might as well send him home. I thought that among familiar surroundings his mind would return quickly to normal.

That's what happened. A day after he was home he was himself again; mentally clear and active, though, of course, still a bit weak from his operation. A few weeks later I injected dye into the tube I had left in Ed's common bile duct and X-rays again showed that there were no stones and that the bile could flow freely into the intestine. I pulled the tube out. (The small hole left in the bile duct usually heals over in a day or two.)

"Seems as if you should be all set now, Ed," I said.

"Great, Doc," he said. "I sure hope so."

Then, to my chagrin, Ed had another attack of pain and jaundice early in March 1978, just three months after his gallbladder operation. Happily, it cleared up spontaneously in three days. "A small stone probably came down from your liver, Ed," I said. "That happens sometimes."

I hoped it wouldn't happen again, but in mid-April 1978, it did. This time, Ed got deeply jaundiced. Other than a poor appetite he didn't feel badly so I tried to "ride it out," hoping the stone would pass, but it didn't.

"Damn it, Ed," I said, "it looks as if we're going to have to open you up again. I've been hoping you'd pass the stone as you apparently did in March, but you've been jaundiced now for almost two weeks, and I'm

afraid if I don't operate soon you'll develop trouble
from all that bile backing up into your liver."

"I hate the idea, Doc, but if it has to be, it has to be. I
can't go on like this. My appetite is shot and I'm losing
a lot of weight. It makes me weak. I don't even feel up
to playing golf."

On April 25, 1978, I again operated on Ed. The
operation was a difficult, tedious one, as is any reop-
eration on the common bile duct. There's always a lot of
scar tissue to go through and it's often difficult even to
find the duct. The surgeon has to be very careful so that
he doesn't cut any essential blood vessels, particularly
those carrying blood to the liver. These blood vessels
run just behind and to one side of the bile duct; in fact,
in second operations, the vessels are usually stuck right
on the duct. This was the situation in Ed's case.

The operation took about two hours. After cleaning
sludge out of the duct—there weren't any solid stones in
it—I used an instrument to stretch the lower end in the
hope that I would never again have to operate on Ed. I
flushed the duct out a dozen times, trying to wash out
any stones that might be up in the liver. I had done this
during the previous operation—it's a routine part of an
exploration of a common bile duct—but this time I was
extremely vigorous. After putting in another T-tube,
getting X-rays which again showed good flow into the
bowel and didn't show any stones in the duct, I closed
the incision. I'd operated through my old incision and
so this time, instead of using buried silk stitches as I
customarily do, I closed with big wire ones that pulled
together all the layers of the abdominal wall in one unit.
I was afraid the stress of these repeated operations
might be taking a toll on Ed's ability to heal, and the
wire sutures would give his wound extra support.

After his usual, confused postoperative convalescence, I sent Ed home where, again, he quickly regained
his alertness. In fact, for some reason, he bounced back
from this third operation even more rapidly than he had

from the second. When I pulled his T-tube on the 16th of June he said, "I don't know why, Doc, but I have a feeling we've finally got this thing licked." Strangely, I shared his optimism.

As I said at the beginning of the chapter, I last saw Ed when he was finishing a round of golf in August, two months after his third major operation. In April 1979 he turned ninety and according to Harold, who sees him occasionally if Ed gets a cold or some minor ache, Ed feels just great. He goes to the Kiwanis luncheons almost every Wednesday and is looking forward to the golf season.

Nothing miraculous involved in Ed's case, I suppose, except that he's a perfect example of just how hardy at least some of us human beings are. To have gone through three major operations after the age of eighty-six, and to have not only survived them but to have managed to still be alert, active and thriving after ninety is a demonstration of the best of which we are capable.

I think in Ed's case, and most doctors will tell you this about their elderly patients, that the fact that Ed has made an effort to keep up with what's going on in the world and in our local community—has continued to garden, bowl, golf and stay physically active—have all contributed to his total, general good health.

God gives us all bodies and minds. If we're going to keep them in good working condition over the years, keep them strong enough so that they can resist disease and function well, we've got to exercise them. Ed needed some surgical help when, unfortunately, he developed his stomach cancer and gallstone problems, but the vigorous style in which he has led his long life did more to pull him through these crises than the pills and scalpel I used to help him.

I don't even know who first said, "God helps those who help themselves," but in matters of health I think that's certainly true.

12

Sometimes Only Time Can Tell

I hadn't planned to put any "down" cases in this book but I think in this chapter, which deals with head injury victims, it's appropriate to include the stories of two people—a man and a woman—because it's the contrast in the outcome of the cases that makes the point I want to emphasize; how difficult it is to predict what will happen to patients who suffer damage to the brain. Of all the organs in our body, the brain is the one about which we know the least.

It isn't that we haven't studied it. We have. And we've learned a great deal. We know what areas are responsible for certain activities; we have a rough idea of how impulses are transmitted, chemically and electrically, from brain cells out along the spinal cord to the nerves which run to our muscles and enable us to move our arms, hands, legs—all the parts of our body which are under our voluntary control.

We know less about the "autonomic" nervous system, that portion of the system that regulates our heartbeat, our digestive system, the sweat glands that help control our temperature. We can find and even operate on the larger branches of this network of nerves—occasionally we will remove a portion of the autonomic (or "sympathetic") nervous system to prevent excessive reflex spasm in the vessels that supply blood to our limbs—but, for the most part, this autonomic nervous system is truly autonomous and we have little control over it.

When we begin to consider consciousness, memory, logic, and thinking, we get into virtually unexplored territory. In John Stewart Collis' recent, fine book, *Living with a Stranger; A Discourse on the Human Body*, he writes: "This organ, the brain, differs [from other parts of the body] in that it embodies an element or principle not to be found elsewhere in the framework. We call it mind. If we eat brains for lunch, just as we might eat a lamb chop, we do not feel that we are lunching on a piece of mind. But mind has been part of it. We do not know what consciousness is. That mystery has not yet been solved. I am in great hopes that it never will be, for I can't see exactly how cortex could examine the cortex nor thinking have a look at thinking." I applaud Mr. Collis for saying all this so nicely.

But we physicians, in our practices, are not allowed the luxury of philosophizing and then turning our attention to other matters. We are certainly aware that the brain is a mysterious and vital organ. In this era of heart-lung machines and organ transplantation, we have even reached the point where we now define death in terms of brain function; if the brain is dead as determined by electroencephalograms and related criteria, then the patient is dead, even if we can keep the heart and lungs functioning using "supportive" machinery. We treat brain-injured patients as vigorously as we can in the hope that their brain function will return to normal or near normal. But only in retrospect can we tell whether our efforts in specific instances have been wise. The cases of Cecelia and Charlie are examples of the dilemma we often face.

Cecelia Hayes is a tall, slender redhead, now forty years old. She and her husband Tom have lived in Litchfield all their lives. They own and manage a restaurant, which Tom bought from his parents, in a small town north of Litchfield. They have two children, a boy, nine, and a girl, eleven. Until three years ago they were a very happy family.

Then, disaster struck. Cecilia was driving through Litchfield one afternoon, on her way to the restaurant, when her car was hit by a truck. Cecelia was thrown from her car and sustained multiple cuts and bruises along with a severe blow to her head.

Lou Fisher, one of our local G.P.s, was called to the hospital to see her and he in turn called me. Cecelia was unconscious and her pupils were fixed, which means they didn't open and close in response to light. However, she did respond to pain by moving her extremities and she was breathing regularly.

After getting X-rays, which showed no evidence of a skull fracture, we took Cecelia to the operating room. Under a very light general anesthetic we sewed up all her cuts, one of which went down to the skull and ran across most of the top of her head. Then we did a tracheotomy on her. A tracheotomy is a procedure in which a curved metal or plastic tube is inserted into the windpipe (the trachea) through an incision in the lower part of the neck. There are a lot of reasons for doing a tracheotomy; it can, for example, be life-saving in a patient who is choking to death on a piece of food lodged in his windpipe. We did the tracheotomy on Cecelia because she was unconscious and we felt that it would help us keep her breathing under control and her airway clear until she woke up. We knew that might not be necessary—possibly she'd be wide awake in another hour—but we couldn't be sure. There's a rule in medicine which says, "When you start thinking that perhaps you ought to do a tracheotomy, do it. Otherwise, when it becomes obvious you need one, it may be too late." So we did the procedure. If it proved to be unnecessary, we could simply pull the tube out after a couple of days and the incision would heal over. But in the meantime we would be able to make certain Cecelia got all the oxygen she needed.

Unfortunately Cecelia didn't wake up in two hours. Nor did she wake up in two days. By then we had had an electroencephalogram done which showed some brain activity, but not a normal pattern. Her pupils were still fixed—a sign of severe brain damage—and she still responded slightly to painful stimuli. In other words, she hadn't changed much.

For three days we gave her intravenous feedings. Then, since she couldn't eat in her unconscious state, we passed a Levin tube through her nose into her stomach and started feeding her fluids through that.

During these first few hours and days we talked regularly and frequently with her husband and children. We kept them fully appraised of her condition but when they'd ask, "Is she going to die?" or "When will she wake up?" we had no answers. We simply did not know.

Ten days after Cecelia had been admitted with her head injury her condition remained unchanged. We had repeated the electroencephalogram, and the brain waves were no different than they had been. Her heartbeat and blood pressure were fine; she breathed on her own, regularly and adequately; she still moved her arms slightly when we pinched very hard.

Two weeks after admission we took her back into the operating room. This time, again under a very light anesthetic—because she would move a little in response to pain if we hadn't used one—we made a small incision in her abdomen and put a catheter, a wide rubber tube about an inch in diameter, into her stomach. We brought the other end directly out through her abdominal wall. We did this operation because the nurses could then squirt baby food directly into her stomach and we were able to remove the Levin tube. If you leave that sort of tube in place for more than two or three weeks, it causes irritation of the lining of the nose and throat and may trigger hemorrhages. Besides, a tube passed through the nose is never big enough to allow passage of the bulky food that ought to be given a patient who will need tube feedings for a long while, and we were naturally beginning to wonder if Cecelia was falling into that category. Which, as you've probably guessed, she did.

Three years have now elapsed and Cecelia still lies in bed unconscious. Her physical condition hasn't changed appreciably since the day she came in. Nor has her electroencephalogram or any of her neurological findings. The nurses squirt baby food into her stomach tube every four hours, they move her arms and legs to keep the joints from stiffening, and they collect her urine from a catheter that we inserted in her bladder early in the course of her injury. Her bowels move spontaneously once or twice a day.

Tom or one of her parents usually comes in to see her every other day or so, but there is really nothing to do but look at her. It's as if she's in a deep sleep.

She is not like Karen Quinlan. I, as a physician, don't have to concern myself about turning off the machinery that keeps Cecelia alive, because there's no machinery to turn off. Her brain is obviously damaged, but the part of the brain that keeps her lungs breathing and her heart beating is working fine. I suppose I could tell the nurses to stop feeding her and, eventually, she'd starve to death. But I wouldn't give that order and if I did the nurses wouldn't follow it. Cecelia's insurance ran out after the first year in the hospital. Now welfare pays about sixty dollars a day for her care in a local nursing home. A doctor makes a routine visit to her once a month, but there's nothing I or any other doctor can do to help her.

Cecelia may go on like this for another ten years or more; she is a very strong woman. On the other hand, she may develop pneumonia or a bad bladder infection, at which time I will have to decide whether to treat her with antibiotics or just ignore the infection and hope she dies of it. If you asked me right now what I'll do if that situation arises, I'll tell you, honestly, I don't know; I'll decide at the time. My guess is that I'll treat the infection, at least the first time it occurs; I may not treat it if it comes a second time. Who knows?

Is it still possible, three years after her injury, that Cecelia will "wake up?" Yes, it is. Not likely, but possible. I have a forty-five year old patient right now, in December 1979, who sustained a severe head injury almost five years ago when he fell off his garage roof. I'll call him Roger. Until September 1979, Roger was just as unresponsive as Cecelia. However, over the last three months, we've been able to remove his gastrostomy tube because he can now swallow and can be fed by the nurses. He is starting to regain the use of his arms; five weeks ago he started pushing himself in a wheelchair. He can't walk yet but just last week the physiotherapist in the nursing home where he stays told me that Roger stood and took a few steps, with help, in a walker. He hasn't spoken yet, but he has started to make sounds that resemble words. It is possible that he'll come back, possibly nearly to normal.

Ask any neurologist or neurosurgeon of experience and I'm sure they'll be able to tell of several patients much like Roger who have made almost complete recoveries. The brain is an amazing organ. To give up prematurely on its chances of recovering from an injury would be, to put it kindly, extremely presumptuous.

Anyway, at this point I have no decisions to make; Cecelia has become a part of the nursing home. We think of her as a patient, of course; she doesn't really look any different than the day she came in. But we treat her more like a vegetable that needs watering and feeding than like a human. That, in fact, is what she's doing: vegetating. And there isn't anything I or anyone else can do about it.

Now, before you make up your mind about the propriety of the care I gave and am giving Cecelia, let me tell you about Charlie.

I first saw Charlie at about three o'clock on a Thursday afternoon. Coincidentally, it was just four days after Cecelia was admitted to the hospital.

Charlie was a patient of Pete Meredith, a family practitioner. He called from the hospital and said, "Bill, come on over, will you? I've got a guy in here with a bad head injury and I could use a consultation." I was at the hospital in five minutes; you can get from any one point in Litchfield to any other in that time, unless you're held up by a train passing through town.

By the time I arrived Charlie was in the intensive care unit. Chuck Fuller, our anesthetist, was there too, and he had put an endotracheal tube, a hollow plastic tube through which air and/or oxygen can be pumped into the lungs, into Charlie's windpipe. Charlie was breathing only because the respirator was breathing for him.

"What's the story, Pete?" I asked.

"Charlie's sixty-three," Pete said. "I saw him in the office just yesterday when he came in with a pain in his shoulder; just a mild case of bursitis. He was slightly drunk at the time. I told him to take some aspirin, put a heating pad on the shoulder and take it easy for a few days. Charlie works as a hired man on a farm three miles west of town.

"Today he'd had a few drinks and when he was driving into town, he went off the road and hit a tree. When the ambulance got to him he was still breathing on his own, but he stopped on the way to the hospital and one of the rescue squad gave him artificial respiration. Chuck happened to be in the hospital when they brought Charlie in and, as you can see, he slipped an endotracheal tube in and put him on the respirator. They've taken some skull films which should be here shortly."

When the X-rays arrived a few minutes later they showed a fracture at the back of the skull, presumably where Charlie had hit the tree. He had a couple of cuts on his arm and he also had a broken right femur (the big bone in the thigh). The fracture of the femur was displaced, but not too badly.

I examined Charlie, as had Pete, and neither of us could find any evidence of hemorrhage inside the skull. When someone has a head injury the doctor looks for what we call "lateralizing" signs, in other words, evidence that there is bleeding on one side of the brain or the other. Lateralizing signs include such things as one pupil being larger than the other, abnormal reflexes or one side but not the other, or inability to move the extremities on one side but not the other. If a patient has lateralizing signs it often means hemorrhage, and angiograms—special X-rays in which dye is injected into the blood vessels to the brain—are done. If they confirm the diagnosis then, usually, you operate and try to stop the bleeding.

Since we couldn't find any lateralizing signs we figured that Charlie, like Cecelia, had generalized brain damage—bruising and/or swelling—and that the proper treatment would be to give him medicine which could, hopefully, reduce the swelling. (We'd also give this to Cecelia.) The drugs we use include diuretics, which increase fluid excretion, and decadron, which is similar to cortisone, but, in some way which is not completely understood, has a rapid, marked effect on reducing swelling of the brain. Then we'd keep him under close observation, checking his neurological findings at frequent intervals. (Actually the nurses in the intensive care unit would do most of the checking, but one of the doctors would examine Charlie three or four times a day, at least for the first few days.) Should lateralizing signs develop, then we'd transfer him to Minneapolis to the care of a neurosurgeon. We knew when she came in that Cecelia was in bad shape and unlikely to survive;

Charlie seemed to be even more severely injured.

I said to Pete, "Why don't you call Jim Roberts and tell him about Charlie, just in case he has any suggestions?" Jim Roberts is the specialist to whom we refer most of our neurosurgical cases. "I suppose I might as well," Pete said, "but I doubt he'll have anything else to offer."

While Pete made the phone call I helped the nurse put traction on the broken femur. Ordinarily, if the fractured femur were Charlie's only problem, I'd have operated and put a pin into the bone to hold it in place. But his head injury was obviously a bad one and took precedence over the fracture. To operate on his leg wouldn't have been reasonable. Actually, I didn't think Charlie would last more than twenty-four hours; but if I were wrong, and he should live, I could operate later. And if I didn't operate the femur would probably heal in two or three months anyway.

When Pete had finished talking to Jim Roberts he came back to the bedside. "Jim says it sounds as if Charlie would be racking up his cue very soon." (Doctors have a lot of euphemisms for "dying.") "He agrees with the way we plan to manage him. May as well go home."

Two days later Charlie's condition was unchanged, so I took him into the operating room and put in a tracheotomy. Charlie was so far under that we didn't need any anesthesia to operate on his neck. He still wasn't breathing on his own. I still didn't think it would be reasonable to operate on the femur. For that we'd have needed anesthesia to relax the thigh muscles, and I thought anesthesia would kill Charlie.

After another week, as I had with Cecelia, I did a gastrostomy on Charlie so we could feed him baby food.

"Damn," I said to Pete at the time, "two hopeless cases in one week. What a cheery business we're in."

Then, three weeks after he'd been admitted to the

hospital, I came into the intensive care unit one morning to see Charlie and Miss Owens, the nurse, said, "He's beginning to fight the respirator, Dr. Nolen. I think he's started to breathe on his own." Sure enough, when we shut the respirator off, after about two minutes Charlie took a couple of breaths. He wasn't breathing deeply or regularly enough to keep himself alive without help, but we shifted the respirator from "constant" to "demand." That meant the respirator would only breathe for Charlie when Charlie didn't breathe for himself.

Over the next two weeks we gradually weaned Charlie off the respirator; five weeks after his accident, he was off it entirely. He had even opened his eyes and he would sometimes respond to simple commands like "squeeze my hand."

Within two months Charlie was wide awake, eating, talking and up in a wheelchair. His femur wasn't solidly healed so we couldn't get him up on crutches, but it was coming along. Three months after he'd come in, virtually dead, Charlie was back at the farm where he lived and worked. He was still on crutches but other than that he was unchanged.

The next time I saw him, about a year after the accident, he was in a local tavern having a few beers.

"Let me buy you a beer, Doc," he said. "You guys sure did a good job on me." I had one with him.

Actually, as ought to be apparent, we really hadn't done much; just the few simple things it took to keep Charlie alive and reasonably well till his brain swelling went away and the bruises healed. But no one would have predicted, when Charlie came in, that he'd recover completely. I'd have bet that Charlie would, as Jim Roberts predicted, "rack up his cue," and I'd have also bet that Cecelia would have at least awakened and, possibly, made it back to normal a few months after she came in. I'd have been wrong in both cases.

What will I do the next time a brain-injured patient is brought to our hospital and put under my care? I'll do exactly as I did in both Cecelia and Charlie's cases. I'll work as hard as I can, utilizing every tool we have available, to keep that patient alive in the hope that hours, days, weeks or months later he or she will recover, as Charlie did. Only when there is absolutely no evidence of brain activity—when I am certain my patient is technically dead—will I unplug the respirator and end the pseudo-life of my patient.

As a physician I have no choice but to fight as hard as I can for the life of anyone under my care. But with brain-injured patients, perhaps to an even greater extent than with others, the decision as to whether they will or will not survive will depend not on me but on the intrinsic strength of the patient and, if you wish, on God.

13

A Miracle?

In 1969 Ellen Thayer was fifty-two years old.
Ellen has always been a very handsome woman. She's
slender—about 5'10" and always between 125 and 130
pounds. Her husband, Joe, three years older than Ellen,
works as a farm implements dealer. Ellen is a minister
of one of the fundamentalist churches with a small
congregation; there are many such churches in this part
of the midwest. Ellen is a dedicated, religious person,
but not the kind who is so enthusiastic that she tries to
convert you every time she sees you. In fact, she often
kids me, because I'm not overly religious. "Come down
to our church some Sunday, Bill," she'll say, "we'll do
what we can to save you, though I predict it will be a difficult job." Then she laughs; she knows that, as far as
religion is concerned, she and I will always agree to
disagree. She and Joe have three children. In 1969, the
children, two boys and a girl, were all in their late teens.

Ellen came to my office in November for her annual
checkup. "I feel just fine, Bill," she said, "but Joe
always insists that I have these annual examinations. I
suppose it's not a bad idea. Anyway, if it keeps Joe
happy I'm willing to cooperate."

"Now that you're over fifty, Ellen," I said, "I'm inclined to agree with Joe. You ought to have a relatively
complete physical every couple of years and a Pap

smear once a year. If you're feeling well I think once every two years is often enough." I asked Ellen the usual questions about her health and learned that she had no symptoms to suggest that she might be ill. She has always been a busy person, running the church as well as managing her home and family. She seemed to thrive on her demanding schedule. I included in my general physical a pelvic examination and I took a Pap smear from her cervix (which was later reported as normal). Then I did a rectal examination and found, to my surprise, that there was a mass about two inches in circumference high in the rectum, just at the tip of my finger. I told Ellen what I had felt and asked her again about any bowel symptoms, particularly whether or not she had noticed any blood when she had a bowel movement. "No," she said, "nothing like that. I've been perfectly fine."

"Well," I said, "I think I'd better do a proctoscopy and see what this lump looks like. I'll probably take a biopsy—snip off a small piece—if I can reach it. The proctoscopy will be a bit uncomfortable but you won't feel the biopsy. The lining of the bowel and rectum is insensitive to pain."

"Will you do the proctoscopy and biopsy right now?" she asked.

"Might as well," I said, "we have the equipment here in the office and your rectum is empty. The sooner we do it, the sooner we'll know what it is. Probably it's just a polyp, a benign growth, but there's always a possibility it might be a cancer. Then we'd have to do a bigger operation to make certain we cure you."

Ellen agreed with my plan, so I did the proctoscopy —passed a metal tube about one and a half inches in diameter and ten inches long into her rectum and lower intestine. The lump was on the back wall of the rectum about four inches above the anal opening. It was a rather unusual-looking growth about two inches in circumference with a wide base. I used a cutting forceps to bite a piece out of it to send to the pathologist. The biopsy site bled, but not very much.

I told Ellen what I'd seen. "It doesn't look like a typical polyp, but it didn't look like a cancer either. We'll just have to wait for the pathologist's report. I'll tell him to call me as soon as he has a diagnosis. I don't like keeping you in suspense but I'm afraid we'll have to wait at least three days, even if I get the specimen to him today. In the meantime you just go ahead with your regular schedule. You may have a little blood in your stool for the next day or so but there won't be much. Don't worry about it."

Three days later the pathologist called to tell me that the growth was a carcinoid, a relatively rare tumor. They're found occasionally in the stomach, the appendix, the small intestine and—as in Ellen's case—in the rectum. They are a form of cancer but are usually low-grade and slow-growing. Usually the patient can be cured simply by removing the tumor. It isn't necessary to take a wide margin of normal tissue as is the general policy in treating the more malignant forms of cancer.

Some carcinoids, however, do spread widely and behave like high-grade malignant tumors. The cells of these carcinoids get into the bloodstream, spread to other organs and produce odd symptoms such as hot, flushing attacks. Fortunately these malignant carcinoids are relatively rare. I thought it was unlikely that Ellen's carcinoid was one.

I explained all this to Ellen and Joe and then arranged to have her admitted to the hospital the following Monday. She didn't want to miss her Sunday church service and I didn't think a few extra days' delay would make any difference. So on the first Monday in December Ellen came into the hospital. The next day we took X-rays of her stomach and intestine, just to make certain she didn't have another tumor (she didn't) and I scheduled her operation for Thursday morning. I planned to give her a general anesthetic and then, using

a snare, to try removing the entire growth through the
proctoscope. If I couldn't manage to get the entire
tumor using that approach, then I'd open her abdomen,
free up the rectum, and remove the tumor from above.
I'd talked the case over with a friend of mine who
specializes in diseases of the colon and rectum and this
was the plan he felt was most reasonable.

About 1:15 Thursday morning I got a call from the
nurse on the night shift at the hospital. "Dr. Nolen,"
she said, "I wonder if you shouldn't come over and see
Mrs. Thayer. I gave her a sleeping pill at ten-thirty but
about half an hour ago she woke up complaining of
chest pain. She asked for some aspirin and didn't want
me to bother you but this pain worries me. It's right in
the center of her chest and she says it feels as if someone
were pressing on her. She's also complaining of a tight-
ness in her throat. I'm wondering if it might not be a
heart attack."

"That does sound suspicious," I said, "why don't
you call in the lab technician and get an electrocardiogram. I'll be over to see her in a few minutes."

When I arrived I examined Ellen and noticed immediately that she was cold, sweaty and short of breath.
"Sorry to disturb you, Bill," she said.

"Don't worry about me," I said, "it's you I'm concerned about. Tell me about this chest pain."

"It's the strangest thing," she said, "I've never had a
pain in my chest before. This one woke me right out of a
sound sleep. It's almost like a toothache. It's steady and
it sort of bothers me when I swallow. For the last few
minutes I've been having trouble getting a deep breath. I
don't know if this is what they call a heart attack, but it
reminds me of the sort of attacks I've heard about
others having. Maybe it's just preoperation nerves."

"It could be just apprehension," I said, "but let's
make certain. I'm going to listen to your heart and lungs
for a minute." When I did I could hear the crackling
sound known technically as "rales" at the base of each

lung. This is a sign that fluid may be collecting in the lung bases, an early sign of heart failure. The heart rate itself was slightly rapid—about 100 beats a minute where Ellen ordinarily ran about 70 beats—and her blood pressure was down to 90/60 from her normal of 130/84. Everything suggested that she was having a heart attack and was already in early heart failure; i.e., her heart wasn't pumping as effectively as it should have and blood was accumulating in her lungs.

Ellen was usually one of my partner's patients. She had come to me only because her "regular" doctor was on vacation. Since he was still away, and since I don't take care of cardiac patients except in emergencies, I called another of my partners and asked him if he'd mind coming over to see Ellen. By then the lab technician had arrived and the electrocardiogram had been taken. I'm not much good at reading E.K.G.s. I had decided when I was in medical school that I was going to go into surgery, and from that point on had spent very little time studying electrocardiography. My partner came over, I introduced him to Ellen, and after he had examined her and looked at her E.K.G., he said, "It's a little bit early to be definite, Mrs. Thayer, but I think it's very possible you're having a heart attack. I certainly think we'd better postpone your surgery. We'll start you on some medicines to support your heart and we'll give you some nasal oxygen to help your breathing. In the morning we'll repeat your E.K.G. and we'll get some blood tests—tests that are usually abnormal when a patient has heart damage—and we'll see how things are going then. I'm also going to order a hypo for your pain. You'll need your rest."

From that point on, for the next four weeks, my partner took care of Ellen Thayer. I'd drop in and see her every day but I left the management of her heart problem to him. As evidence accumulated—changes in the electrocardiogram together with increases in the blood enzymes (chemicals) that signify death of heart muscle—it was apparent that she had had a heart attack of moderate severity, but she continued to improve steadily. My partner brought her heart failure under control and he gradually increased her activity.

About the middle of the third week I thought I had better discuss the surgery with Ellen. I thought she must be concerned about the delay and I wanted to reassure her. "As far as the tumor in your rectum is concerned," I said, "I don't think you have much to worry about. Of course we'd like to remove it because the longer it stays, the bigger it will become, but this particular variety is almost always very slow-growing. The chance that it will spread beyond the rectum is virtually nil. I think we ought to wait at least eight and maybe ten weeks before we plan to go ahead with the operation. I want to give your heart plenty of time to heal."

"Bill," Ellen said, "I know this is going to sound silly to you but I'm sure of it so I'm going to tell you anyway. There won't be any need for you to operate on that tumor you saw in my rectum. The Lord is going to cure me of it. I can't explain why, but I know He will. Maybe He felt that my heart attack was enough for me to suffer right now. The ways of the Lord aren't always for us to understand. But I am certain as I can be that that tumor is either already gone or it will be when you next look for it."

I really didn't know what to say. I could hardly believe Ellen was right—tumors don't just melt away—but I was reluctant to argue with her. I'd simply wait till the eight weeks were over and reexamine her. (I didn't want to do even a digital examination of her rectum then, let alone a proctoscopy, because stimulation of the rectum occasionally causes reflex stimulation of other organs, including the heart.)

So I waited ten weeks, till Ellen had been home for almost a month, and then called her and asked if she would take a laxative that night and come to my office for a proctoscopy the next day.

"I'll be glad to," she said, "but I'm sure we'll both be wasting our time. The Lord has healed me of that tumor. I sense it."

I couldn't see any point in arguing; I'd have my proof the next day. I just hoped that the tumor hadn't grown significantly.

The next afternoon I examined Ellen. To my very great surprise, when I did a digital examination of her rectum I couldn't feel the tumor. "Maybe," I thought, "I'm just afraid to push too hard."

Then, with my nurse acting as an assistant, Ellen climbed up on the proctoscopy table and I inserted the proctoscope. I passed the proctoscope the full ten inches and saw nothing. I pulled it back to the four-inch marker and looked carefully in the area from which I'd previously taken a biopsy. I couldn't see any abnormality. Not even a puckered scar from the area I had biopsied. I inserted the proctoscope its full length again and once more examined every bit of the lower bowel and rectum; not a trace of the tumor. I helped Ellen get up and, when she was dressed, she came into my office.

"Well," she said, smiling, "when's the operation?"

I smiled back. "Ellen," I said, "there isn't going to be one, as you apparently knew before you came here. That tumor is gone. I'd think I was crazy if I didn't have this biopsy report from the pathologist right here in front of me. Here, look at it yourself. It says clearly 'carcinoid tumor of the rectum.' It was there and now it isn't."

"I don't need to read the report, Bill," she said, "I believe the tumor was there, as you told me. I also knew, as I told you, that God healed me. Read the Bible. I'm not the first one He has healed, and I doubt that I'll be the last."

"I'm in no position to argue with you, Ellen," I said, "not after what's happened. Just do me a favor; come back in three months and let me reexamine you. Not a proctoscopy, just a digital examination. I felt it before

and if it comes back I should be able to feel it again.
Besides, you'll be coming in to see my partner so he can
make sure your heart is coming along nicely. You can
see us both at the same visit.''

"I'll be glad to stop in, Bill," she said, "but don't
worry, it won't come back."

And now, eleven years later, it still hasn't returned.
Ellen continues to work as the minister of her church,
her husband has retired, and her three children are all
living in other parts of the midwest. Ellen, at sixty-
three, is still the same, cheery, vigorous person she was
eleven years ago.

I have no explanation to offer. Cancers have been
known to undergo spontaneous regression. In fact,
there is a book called *Spontaneous Regression of Cancer*, which reports on all the collected cases that have
been documented in the surgical literature. There are
very, very few of them. Possibly this case falls into that
category, though this is the only one I know of in which
the patient predicted, correctly, the cure of a tumor
whose presence had been documented both by visual-
ization and microscopic examination.

There is now a school of thought regarding cancer
that maintains immunity plays a large role. These doctors, most of whom work in cancer centers, believe that
at least occasionally, a patient will develop an immunity
to tumor cells and the healthy cells of his or her body
will reject the cancer cells, often before the cancer is
large enough to be visualized or produce symptoms.
What they are saying, in effect, is that some of us may
have several episodes of cancer during our lifetime but
that, ordinarily, our bodies will fight off these attacks
much as we fight off the viruses and bacteria that assail
us every day. It's only when our immune systems aren't
operating properly that the cancer grows, gets out of
control and may eventually kill us. The doctors who
believe in this immunity theory are hopeful that at some
time we will be able to develop a serum which will give

our bodies specific immunity to cancer; or at least to some forms of cancer, if they are doctors who believe that cancer is not one, but many diseases.

There is, of course, another possible explanation. It may be that God did intervene directly and cure Ellen Thayer of her tumor. My own inclination is to reject that explanation. I like and admire Ellen Thayer. I think she is a remarkable woman. I just don't believe that God (and I use that word in the generally accepted sense) works miracles on an individual basis.

But Ellen Thayer tells me He does and offers her case as an example. I will admit it is as convincing an example as I, who once spent a couple of years unsuccessfully looking for "miracle" cures,* have ever seen.

I had some reservations about writing this chapter. It's potentially dangerous if it's misinterpreted; it might keep patients who need medical care from seeking proper help. I want to be as explicit as possible about the fact that most claims of "miraculous" cures are nonsense. In the two years I spent investigating such claims I found none that could be documented. All were claims made either by charlatans, religious hypocrites, or people who had had either psychosomatic illnesses or self-limited diseases that resolved spontaneously, as most illnesses do.

Perhaps I should emphasize that Ellen Thayer, a very reasonable woman, accepted the standard medical care for her heart attack; that she continues to go to a physician for an annual examination; that she believes, as do I, that all healing may come from God but only in the sense that God created man in His image and gave him a brain to think with and hands to work with so that he could learn how to take care of himself. (I hope no one will be offended that I'm using traditional male ter-

---

* See *Healing: A Doctor in Search of a Miracle*, Random House (1975) and Fawcett (1976).

minology; using "he and she" constantly is simply too wearing.) Ellen believes that in this instance God intervened directly to cure her; I've already expressed my view. But Ellen also feels, as she puts it, that "These roving evangelists who claim to have special healing powers are not only phony, dangerous thieves but reflect very badly on all those who are truly religious and who are members of the organized churches that carry out the day-to-day religious and charitable work that is a necessary part of God's design." To that I can only add, "Amen."

14

Quackery Fails Again

Penny Warta and her husband, Floyd, have been neighbors and friends of ours for all the twenty years we've lived in Litchfield. Floyd taught English in the high school from 1937 till he had to retire at age sixty-five in 1971, but he was best known in the community as the drama teacher. Floyd directed all the school plays, which are well attended by the general public since the nearest theater is seventy miles away in Minneapolis.

Floyd is a big man with a sizable paunch. In fact, a couple of years before he retired he grew a long white beard and, without the need for any padding, quickly became a popular "Santa Claus." Not only did he play the part at various local functions but even became a professional, appearing in television commercials for such sponsors as Arctic Cat, the snowmobile manufacturer. He has continued with his second career as a Santa Claus since his retirement.

Over the years we've been in Litchfield, Penny would occasionally drop in—always after a preliminary phone call—to visit with Joan in the afternoon, often bringing gifts of pastries she'd baked or vegetables Floyd had grown in his backyard garden. They've been fine neighbors, always friendly but never too pushy. (One of the things you have to be wary of in a small town are neighbors who become overly friendly. You find them stopping in every evening. The only cure for such behavior is flagrant rudeness. "Neighborly" neighbors aren't affected by subtleties.)

Penny and Floyd weren't my patients. In a small town it's perfectly possible for people to remain friends with doctors other than the one who is their family physician, just as we doctors remain friends with patients whose businesses we don't patronize. They have been patients of Lennox Danielson for the forty-three years they've lived in Litchfield.

One Wednesday morning in April 1975, Lennox stopped me at the hospital. "Bill," he said, "I've got Penny in the hospital with a huge lump in her left breast. I saw her in the office yesterday and admitted her right away. I'm sure it's a cancer. She admits she's had it for two months but I'll bet she's had it even longer than that.

"I've put her on the schedule for Friday," Lennox continued. "I'm getting a bone scan and a chest X-ray today. If they're negative I suppose we may as well take her breast off. It may be too late to cure her, but if we leave this thing alone it will break down soon, and she'll have a big ulcerating lesion to live with. And, of course, maybe we'll even get lucky and cure her. She's in room three-twenty-four. I told her you'd be stopping in to see her."

About an hour later, after going over both the bone and chest X-rays with the radiologist, who agreed there was no evidence of spread to these places, I went up to Penny's room. When I walked in she said, "Looks like I've been foolish, doesn't it, Bill? I should have gone to Lennox sooner, but I just couldn't bring myself to believe it was anything serious. I kept hoping it would go away."

"Don't worry about that now, Penny," I said. "Lots of women do just as you did, and we cure many of them. Now just lie back, if you don't mind, and let me feel this thing."

Lennox was right, of course. The lump was about the size of a hen's egg. I couldn't feel any enlarged glands in the axilla, but Penny has always been a bit overweight and her fat might well have covered any glands that were enlarged. I told Penny that the lump should be biopsied, that I suspected it was cancer, and that the only reasonable operation for a lump that size was a modified radical mastectomy. I explained the procedure I planned to do and why I thought it appropriate.

Penny said, "Do what you think is proper, Bill. I leave it up to you."

Floyd took the news hard. He blamed himself for the delay in treatment, because he hadn't insisted on annual checkups for Penny. I reassured him—told him Penny had known of the lump for two months and just didn't want to admit it—and that helped him a little. When someone in a family develops a serious disease it's common for other family members—husband, wife, parents—to blame themselves for some action they did or didn't take.

The next day we operated on Penny. The lump was a cancer—a large one—and had spread to five of the twelve bean-shaped lymph nodes I removed from the axilla. When a breast tumor has metastasized (spread) to the axillary nodes the chances of achieving a cure drop by about fifty percent. It was possible we'd cured Penny, but the odds against were about two to one. We explained this to Floyd, who, again, took the news hard. With Penny, Lennox and I were as optimistic as we felt we could honestly be. We assured her we'd removed all the tumor we could find, that there was no definite evidence there was any other cancer in her body, and that many patients with tumors as extensive as hers had been cured. We also explained to both Penny and Floyd that, since some of the glands in the axilla contained tumor, we felt she should have cobalt radiation of her axilla to kill any cancer cells that might have been left behind. When we discharged Penny, two weeks after her operation, we made appointments for her to have cobalt therapy at a hospital near Litchfield, to which she could commute for the two weeks it would take to deliver the proper dosage.

Penny was sixty-nine years old at the time we did the mastectomy in 1975. She tolerated the cobalt treatment without difficulty and was soon back doing her housework, shopping and occasionally visiting Joan. She was cheerful and didn't seem worried about the possibility of a cancer recurrence.

Unfortunately, in June 1978, a little more than three years after her operation, she began to experience back pain. When it hadn't responded to the usual symptomatic treatment—rest, heat and aspirin—she went to see Lennox and he ordered X-rays which showed that the cancer had spread widely to bone. Almost all the vertebrae were involved, as was the pelvis.

Since three years had elapsed without any sign of recurrence they had been very hopeful she was cured. This new development understandably depressed them, and both Penny and Floyd went into a terrible slump.

As we did. We knew now that the chances of curing Penny were extremely slight, but we felt we could at least alleviate her back pain by radiation, and slow down tumor spread either by using hormones, anticancer drugs or both. We explained this to Penny and Floyd and they agreed to the therapy.

At this point one of their very close friends intervened. Laetrile, the friend insisted, was the answer. Penny would be foolish to go through more cobalt therapy and to take in poisonous drugs when Laetrile, together with a special diet, would cure her. Floyd was against the idea, but the friend persuaded Penny. She refused to follow our suggestions for conventional therapy. Lennox reluctantly discharged her, telling her that if she changed her mind she should be certain to phone him.

For the next three months Floyd treated Penny at home. He fed her Laetrile and spent hours every day preparing the special diet prescribed by their friend, the Laetrile/diet advocate. "It was a heck of a tough three months," Floyd said, "but I didn't dare say anything. Penny was so certain it would work that she just about convinced me."

As both Lennox and I expected, the Laetrile/diet therapy did nothing. In fact, on September 9, 1978, after three months of this "treatment," Penny stumbled in her home, struck a glancing blow to her left shoulder, and broke her left humerus; the tumor had now invaded this bone and at the fracture site just a shell of bone remained.

Lennox admitted her to the hospital, applied a plaster splint to the fracture, and put her on pain medicine as necessary. Further X-rays of her bones showed that the tumor had been spreading steadily for the last three months. A check of her blood showed that she was extremely anemic, possibly due in part to bone marrow invasion, but mostly the result of the terrible, malnourishing diet she had been eating.

We told Floyd what the X-rays had shown and he was despondent. "God," he said, "I feel as if I've nearly killed her. I knew I shouldn't have cooperated with that Laetrile business, but Penny insisted. They swore it would make her well."

"Look, Floyd," I said, "don't blame yourself. You did what you felt you had to do. We can't guarantee Penny would have done any better on the therapy we recommended. Sometimes these tumors just won't respond to anything. Now, though, it's time to let us try something other than Laetrile. We know that isn't working."

Floyd agreed and helped us persuade Penny, who was still obstinate. She virtually refused to believe that her condition had deteriorated, despite the Laetrile and diet. But, though she protested, she let us transfuse her and feed her iron supplements and a nutritious diet. Her protests, Lennox and I agreed, were psychologically necessary for her; she couldn't face admitting she'd been wrong.

She was too weak to tolerate the usual anticancer drugs but we started her on female hormone therapy. After a month on this, though her blood level was up near normal as a result of the transfusions, iron and diet, X-rays didn't show any diminution in the extent of the bone metastases. I suggested to Lennox that we discontinue the female hormone therapy and start her on testosterone, a male hormone. Sometimes, for reasons that are still obscure, male hormones work when female hormones won't, though usually, in post-menopausal women (into which category Penny, now seventy-two, fit) female hormone therapy works best.

In Penny's case the testosterone helped. It not only lifted her spirits, a not uncommon effect, but it seemed to speed the healing of her fracture. After two months in the hospital, on November 11, 1978, we were able to discharge Penny to her home.

She was still reluctant to take any other anticancer drugs and we didn't insist; not only because we couldn't guarantee they'd help but because we were afraid if we insisted she'd refuse any therapy at all. We arranged to have a nurse visit Penny's home twice a week to help manage things—she was still weak and limited to a bed-chair life when we discharged her—and we provided the vials of testosterone so that Penny could get a shot of long-lasting testosterone every three weeks.

In March 1979, Lennox told me Floyd and Penny were planning to fly to California the first week of April to visit Penny's sister. "Floyd asked me if I thought it was safe and I told him to go ahead," Lennox said. "Heck, if she's feeling that well she may as well enjoy herself. They made the trip to California and, Floyd told me recently, they had a marvelous time. Floyd is all smiles and Penny seems happy. They never even mention that damn Laetrile anymore, though I think Penny takes some once in awhile, more to satisfy her friend than for any other reason.''

"Great," I said. "It was really heartbreaking to see how depressed they both were when they realized all the time spent on that crazy diet and the money spent on the Laetrile had been wasted. It's probably just as well she broke that arm. Otherwise they'd certainly have continued on that stuff till she died.''

It's now March 1980. Floyd stops in to see me every few weeks and he tells me Penny is stronger every day. She is up most of the time and even walks the few blocks to the town center. She has no pain; her blood level, which we recently checked, remains normal; her spirits are excellent. "Frankly," Floyd said when I saw him last week, "I'm amazed. She looked so terrible when we brought her to the hospital last fall I honestly didn't think she'd ever get out.''

The moral of this story is, I hope, fairly plain. We haven't got an answer to the problem of breast cancer, but every year progress is being made. New anticancer drugs have been developed which, in some studies, have been shown to improve the cure rate for certain patients. These drugs are administered immediately after surgery.

We also know that some patients—Penny is an example—respond remarkably well to hormone therapy. It may not cure the disease but it can arrest it and, in some cases, destroy metastatic tumor for long periods of time. Certainly, there are patients in which the disease becomes so widely disseminated that cure or even arrest is impossible. When that happens the only reasonable course to follow is one of palliation: make the patient as comfortable as possible for as long as possible. But with the new developments in radiation treatment and anticancer drug therapy, such situations are far less likely to occur than was previously the case.

The danger, which Penny's case illustrates, is that patients who develop breast cancer, primary or recurrent, will turn to Laetrile—or to quackery—looking for the quick, miraculous cure that orthodox medicine cannot as yet offer. When and if this happens delay in the application of appropriate therapy may occur, sometimes leading to disaster.

Anyone who believes that the American Medical Association or individual doctors are engaged in a conspiracy to withhold cancer cures from the public might try looking into the obituary column at the back of each weekly issue of the *Journal of the A.M.A.* The reader would find that doctors die of the same diseases as do their patients. The families and friends of physicians also die of these diseases. Why would we conspire to suppress news of a medicine that would save the lives of millions of patients, including our families, our friends, ourselves and members of our own profession? We wouldn't and we don't.

Please avoid quackery; it can easily cost you your life.

15

The Placebo Effect—or Was It?

Frank Smith is a doctor I've met only a few times over the last twenty years, usually at the golf club when he and his wife have been in Litchfield to visit their daughter, son-in-law and grandchildren. Frank is a G.P. in a town I'll call Mount Vernon, about eighty miles north of Litchfield. In the late summer of 1979, as I write this, he has recently turned seventy-five. He retired from his very busy general practice when he was seventy, but he still sees and cares for a few of his long-time patients. "And I visit the nursing home, too," he told me. "A lot of my long-time patients live there and I think at least half the good I do for them is simply the pleasure they get out of having an acquaintance, who knew them when they were young and vigorous, still showing some interest in them."

Frank is a big man—about 6 feet tall and just a bit under 200 pounds—and he is still in good condition. "Now I'm retired, I play golf here in Mount Vernon almost every day in the late spring, summer and early fall. We move to Texas in the winter and I play and swim almost every day down there. I had enough of these Minnesota winters during the forty-five years I was in practice here."

I had driven to Mount Vernon to visit Frank because I'd heard, from his daughter, that back in the early fifties Frank, and just about all the doctors who helped take care of him, didn't think he'd live very long. Then he had an operation on his heart and now, almost thirty years later, he was still going strong. I knew that the heart operations being done in the early 1950's had statistically been proven valueless, so I wanted to know more about Frank's experience. I told Frank that I thought his story might be suitable for the book I was working on and I promised I'd change the details so that he could preserve his anonymity. He was willing to cooperate, so on an August afternoon we sat out in the backyard of his home and, as we sipped iced tea, he told me his story.

"It began in the summer of 1951," he said, "when I was forty-seven years old. My wife, Josie, and I had taken our four children—they ranged in age from eight to seventeen—on a summer vacation out to Yellowstone Park. I hadn't been sick a day in my life, except for minor colds. I think just working hard—as I had to do then, because I was one of only two doctors in Mount Vernon—kept me in good shape. Most of the exercise I got came from running up and down the hospital stairs.

"We were enjoying ourselves, staying at a lodge, fishing and just tramping in the woods, getting the relaxation that I thought I really needed. There was a fair-sized mountain—or maybe you'd just call it a big hill—not far from our lodge, so one day the kids and I thought we'd hike up it. The kids ran ahead but I didn't push myself. I just walked along at a reasonably good pace.

"About halfway up that hill I began to notice a pain in my chest. I thought it might just be a muscle cramp so I kept on going, but the darn thing kept getting worse and after another five minutes I had to stop and rest. When I did the pain went away. I'd taken care of enough cases of heart trouble so that I realized I could be having angina [heart pain caused by insufficient blood supply to the heart muscle, usually caused by arteriosclerosis to the heart], but I found that difficult to believe. My parents had both lived into their eighties, I was in reasonably good shape, and I'd had an electrocardiogram taken just six months earlier as part of an insurance physical, and it was perfectly normal. The pain went away in about three minutes and after I had rested another five minutes I started up the mountain again. It wasn't more than two or three minutes before that darn pain came back, and this time it seemed to me as if my left arm were going numb. I decided I'd better not take any chances. I let the kids finish the climb but I walked back down to the lodge.

"It was angina, all right, and it quickly got worse. I was a smoker—two to three packs a day—and I quit, hoping that would help, but it didn't. After we returned from our vacation I went back to work, but within three months my angina had gotten so bad I couldn't walk more than a hundred steps without an attack of pain. I was eating nitroglycerine tablets [the traditional drug used to relieve the pain of angina] like they were candy. Harold Diamond, the other doctor in town, ran a two-step test on me; you know, where you run up and down two steps while the E.K.G. leads are strapped to you? That test is about obsolete now, with all the fancy stress test machines, but even that old two-step test produced very clear changes in my electrocardiogram. I went down to see a heart specialist, Lou Lester in Minneapolis, and he agreed it was angina. He suggested I take three months off, so I did. Josie and I left the kids with her sister who lives here in Mount Vernon and we went down to Florida. From December till March all I did was lie around in the sun. I didn't even swim much, though I walked about a mile every morning and evening. If I walked very slowly I was all right; as soon as I tried to walk fast I'd get the chest pain. I had to be very careful crossing streets. I'd wait till there was no traffic anywhere near me because I knew that if I had to step fast I might have a coronary. Thank God, even though I had angina I hadn't yet had a real coronary. As far as we could tell my heart muscle was still healthy. It was just that there wasn't room in the coronary arteries to get enough blood to the muscle so that I could exercise. There weren't any angiograms [X-rays of the arteries to the heart] then, so we didn't know where the block or blocks were, but I and all the doctors I'd seen were sure from my symptoms that I was blocked someplace.

"I came back to Minnesota in March 1952 and went back to work, but I wasn't any better; I still had to be careful crossing streets and I plodded up the hospital steps like an old man. As you can imagine, I was getting desperate. I had four youngsters and a wife to support and I'd seen enough patients with progressive angina, like mine, to know the chances were excellent that one day soon I was going to have a coronary and that could well be the end of me."

Frank paused for a moment. "Sure I'm not boring you?" he asked.

"Not at all," I said. "I'm anxious to hear what happened."

"Let me get us a little more iced tea and I'll finish the story," he said, getting up and strolling into the house. With his silvery hair and his trim, erect posture, he looked closer to sixty-five than seventy-five. A couple of minutes later he was back and he continued his story.

"About two weeks after I'd gotten back, about the middle of March, I got a call one evening from Dr. Lester [all names in this chapter have been changed], the cardiologist in Minneapolis who was following my case. 'Frank,' he said, 'can you come down to Minneapolis the day after tomorrow? There's a surgeon visiting here from out east—he operated on a mitral valve today —and I've told him about your case. There's a new operation for angina that's supposed to increase the blood flow to the heart. Claude Beck, the surgeon in the midwest who thought it up, has had a lot of luck doing it on dogs, but of course the anatomy in dogs is different than it is in humans, and supposedly the doctors on the staff of his hospital are reluctant to let him do it on humans. The doctor here is from the northeast. His name is Jake Gans. You've probably heard of him because he's been leading the way in the development of heart surgery. He believes the operation this midwesterner developed has merit. He's done some on humans—at the hospital where he works they let him do pretty much what he wants, since he's begun to have success with this mitral valve procedure—and if after he examines you he still considers you a good candidate, I think you might be wise to go out east and have the operation done.' I tell you I jumped at the chance to go to Minneapolis and see this fellow Gans. I was desperate for some help.

"On Thursday, Josie and I drove to Minneapolis and spent the night at a hotel. I wanted to be well rested when I saw Dr. Gans the next morning. At ten o'clock I was over at Lou Lester's office and he introduced me to Gans. Gans was an affable fellow—big, broad smile, strong handshake, looked like he thought there was nothing in the world he couldn't do. Frankly, that's the kind of an attitude I like in a doctor, particularly a surgeon. If he isn't cocky—and Gans was certainly cocky—then I'm afraid he lacks confidence in himself, and if there's anything a patient doesn't need it's an insecure surgeon.

"Lou Lester had given him a complete rundown on my history and they'd reviewed my electrocardiogram together. Gans examined me, asked a few questions about the nature of my pain, and then said, 'Dr. Smith, you're walking through a mine field every minute of every day. You know it and I know it. Any one of these angina attacks could signal a complete block of one of your coronary arteries and that might be the end. Otherwise you're in good shape. There's no doubt in my mind. I think we ought to operate on you and improve the circulation to your heart.' "

"Gans wasn't a fellow to pull punches, was he," I asked.

"No," Frank replied, "and I respected him for it. I knew I was in trouble and there was no sense pretending I wasn't. I didn't hesitate. Three days later I flew back to Mercy Hospital where he was chief of surgery. One of the cardiologists on Gans's staff checked me over, agreed I needed the operation, and it was scheduled for the twenty-eighth of March."

"What operation was it?" I asked.

The one they called the Beck Two. Gans did it in two stages. During the first stage, he removed a superficial vein from my arm, opened my chest, sewed one end to the aorta and the other end to the coronary sinus, which he only partly tied off; apparently he didn't want to put too much sudden strain on the small veins that would have to take over when the coronary vein was completely tied off. I expect you're up-to-date on heart anatomy, but in case you aren't, the coronary sinus is the big vein that drains blood from the left ventricle veins and empties that blood into the right atrium. [The ventricles are the muscular, pumping portions of the heart; the atria are the collecting sacs of the heart into which blood from all the organs of the body, including the lungs, flows.] If you tie off the coronary sinus, then other small veins in the four chambers of the heart will dilate and drain the blood that reaches the heart muscle. The heart is the only organ in the body where the anatomy is such that a maneuver like this is possible. What Gans was doing was turning the coronary sinus into an artery, which he hoped would help nourish the heart.

"Three weeks later, about the 20th of April, he opened my chest again and tightened up the sutures so that the coronary vein now acted completely as an artery. One week later I was home and two months later, on the first of July, I was back at work. I rarely had any discomfort in my chest and felt like my old self again. My electrocardiogram showed some minor changes when I took the two-step test, but nothing nearly as bad as before the operation. I was able to keep practicing twenty-three more years, till the kids were grown and I was seventy. I could have kept going after that but, to tell the truth, I'd had enough. I'm happy to be able to sit around and relax now."

"You know," I said, "that most investigators felt the Beck Two operation didn't do any more to improve the circulation to the heart than did the Beck One." (In the Beck One, described by Dr. Claude Beck in 1935, the heart was exposed and the surface was abraded, and sometimes a talcum powder irritant was applied to its surface in hope that this irritation would stimulate the formation of new blood vessels to the heart.)

"I know that," Frank replied. "I realize that the operation fell into disrepute because no one could ever prove that it actually improved circulation.

"I also realize that a lot of my friends assume that my chest pain was probably psychological and that my relief was obtained through a placebo effect. [Placebo means "I will please" in Latin, and a "placebo" effect is said to have occurred when a patient's symptoms are relieved or disappear after the patient has been given a pill known to contain only ingredients that can't possibly play anything but a psychological role in relieving the patient's symptoms. So-called "sugar pills" are the most common placebos but an operation done to relieve symptoms may, and often does, have a placebo effect. If, for example, the patient had a hernia or a tumor—something that can be seen—then a placebo operation, in which only a skin incision is made, would be obviously ineffective.] I've stopped arguing with them, since there's no way I can prove that the operation actually improved the circulation to my heart. What I can say is this. I have always been considered an emotionally stable person, not given to complaining about pain unless it was severe. In 1951 I developed severe, progressive pain typical of angina, and I did everything I could, medically, to relieve it. I didn't get any better. The electrocardiogram showed the changes typically caused by angina.

"I underwent a relatively new operation of unproven value because I didn't want to live with this pain any longer; and both my cardiologist and I thought I would die if I couldn't get that circulation improved. I knew the operation was risky; Gans told me, before he operated, that eight of his first thirteen patients had died. But he also told me that those who died were elderly, very ill, poor-risk patients—about the only kind a surgeon ever gets to operate on when he's trying to prove the value of a new operation—and that he thought, given my general condition, I could survive the operation and be improved by it. I underwent those operations knowing very well that I was taking a chance and that I might not survive.

"Three months after those operations I was a well man and I've remained well ever since. I think the operation improved the circulation to my heart; I *know* that following the operation I no longer had disabling angina. Now if someone wants to say that it was the psychological effect of having my chest opened twice that relieved my angina, I can't argue with him, since I have no way of proving what actually went on in my heart muscle after Gans hooked the aorta to the coronary sinus. Maybe if there's an autopsy after I die, the answer will be clear. But I'm in no hurry to prove that point one way or another.

"I can certainly say I'm awfully glad I decided to have the operation. I've enjoyed, and continue to enjoy, my life. Twenty-eight years ago, when I was disabled by that angina, I wondered if I'd be lucky enough to live another year. Now I've seen my children grow up and am enjoying my grandchildren—in small doses, of course, as grandchildren should be enjoyed. I have a nice life.''

There have been, over the last fifty years, innumerable operations designed to relieve angina. Along with the Beck One and Two we've gone through eras where the lung or the omentum (the fatty apron that hangs from the stomach) were sutured to the heart; years when the nerves to the heart were being divided, to relieve pain; a time when the thyroid gland was removed in the hope that by removing thyroid hormone, which stimulates the heartbeat, strain would be taken off the heart; operations of all sorts were done, none of which—including the Beck Two—stood the test of time. None could be proven to be of more value than a sham operation or possibly, a placebo pill. (The latest operation, the coronary bypass, in which veins are used to bridge obstructed areas in the arteries to the heart after they have been visualized on X-ray, seems to me, after a thorough review of the literature, to be efficacious not only in relieving angina but in prolonging life. Since I had such an operation in 1975, and have lived an active, angina-free life since that time, I am, admittedly, prejudiced. But after reviewing ten years of collected experience, the value of the operation seems to me beyond dispute, though not all doctors agree.)

However, the point of writing Frank's story is not to lead to a discussion of the merits of specific heart operations. Instead I've related Frank's story, as he told it to me, because it demonstrates so well how often the boundaries between psychological and physical problems are unclear. Some doctors would argue that Frank's story demonstrates only that the placebo effect is often a powerful one; that, attaching the aorta to the coronary sinus was no more useful in improving heart circulation than a sham operation—simply incising the skin—would have been.

To which increasing numbers of doctors are now

saying, so what? Admittedly, if a doctor knew an operation wasn't going to offer anything but psychological relief to a patient, he should do only the minimal, low-risk operation necessary to achieve that effect; perhaps making a short skin incision in the chest wall, which could be done with virtually no mortality. In Frank's case, at the time, no one knew for certain that the Beck Two operation wasn't any better than a sham procedure. (There are still some doctors who will argue that the Beck Two did, indeed, improve circulation in some hearts; but they are few in number and have never been able to prove their case. In any event, the coronary bypass operation—which wasn't possible in 1951, since at that time we didn't have reliable heart-lung machines or X-ray techniques to outline the coronary arteries—is universally agreed to be much sounder in principle and more effective in results than any previous operation for the relief of angina.)

But the entire morality and reasonableness of using placebos is again being ardently discussed. Assume, for example, that after you give a harmless "sugar pill" to a patient that patient reports her pain is gone. Have you done any harm? Doctors, I among them, would answer "no." We know that many common problems—ulcers of the duodenum and stomach, asthma, migraine and tension headaches, menstrual cramps, ulcerative colitis; the list is virtually endless—often have a psychological as well as a physiological or anatomical cause. If a placebo—which is completely harmless—brings relief to, say, forty percent of these patients (a figure frequently attainable), then why not try using it rather than some other potent drug, which might relieve, say, ninety percent of patients. The placebo should not only be very inexpensive but should not cause any undesirable side effects; neither claim can be made for most "standard" medications.

In the sixty percent of patients in which the placebo isn't effective, the doctor can switch to the more potent, and more expensive and dangerous, drugs.

No one really knows why placebos work. To say they only work on patients whose problems are "all in their head" is usually considered a disparaging description. But perhaps we should take the remark literally and seriously. It may be that the patient's psyche will be so modified by the placebo that her mind will affect her body in a manner that will relieve the pain and/or cure the disease. This is not an unreasonable assumption, since—as I've already noted—migraines, ulcers, etc. are often caused by psychological problems ("nervous tension," to use the common phrase) and we know that the mind, working through the nervous system, can affect the body. Perhaps the placebo stimulates the nervous system to produce positive, healing effects instead of painful, destructive ones.

When we know more—much more—about the brain and the mind (we're not yet even specifically clear how the two are related), then we may be able to use placebos more scientifically than we now do. But in the meantime placebo treatment seems to me to deserve a far larger place in the doctor's armamentarium than it now enjoys.

Frank Smith, with whom I discussed this placebo problem at some length, agrees. As he says, "Whether the operation was a placebo or not doesn't bother me. I'm just damn glad I had it. One way or another it has given me twenty-eight years of enjoyable life I wouldn't otherwise have had."

16

Cured . . . We Hope

In August 1971, Judy Rankin, a housewife/real estate saleswoman, came to my office on a Tuesday afternoon. Judy was then thirty-three, the mother of two children: Lisa, four, and Frankie, two. Judy's husband, Leo Rankin, taught high-school physics and chemistry in a small town a few miles from Litchfield.

Judy is about 5' 10'' tall, has long blond hair, and is very attractive. She is stocky but not fat, muscular and well coordinated. She is an excellent tennis player and my wife, Joan, and I had played mixed doubles with Judy and Leo many times during the five years they had lived in Litchfield. I always played with Judy, and Leo and Joan were partners. Joan and I both agree we ought never, ever to play either bridge or tennis as partners if we intend to remain married. Like most husbands I am far more tolerant of my partner's errors if my partner is not my wife. (It has been said by many of our tennis opponents that Joan generally makes many fewer errors than do I, but I pay no attention to such ridiculous statements.)

Judy apologized as soon as she was shown into my office. "I know you don't do general practice, Bill," she said, "but since we're friends—and since, frankly, I'm very frightened—I thought you wouldn't mind if I came in to see you first. If it's necessary you can refer me to another doctor.''

"Don't apologize, Judy," I said, "I'm always glad to see you. Just sit down and relax and tell me what's bothering you. Then we'll decide what has to be done."

She sat down, breathed a sigh of relief, and said, "Gee, it will be good just to tell this story to someone. I haven't even told Leo yet. You know what a worrier he is. I didn't want to frighten him unnecessarily.

"It began two days ago. I was playing tennis with Helen Fogarty—you know what a patty-caker she is, I can usually blow her off the court—but halfway through the second set my game began to fall apart. I remember distinctly the very first thing that went wrong. Helen hit a lob, not a very good one, and I moved in to smash it. But when I started to swing I found I was seeing double. It looked like two balls were coming down at me. I hit at what I guessed was the real ball but it went off the side of my racket out of the court. Helen laughed and so did I. It was hot two days ago. We were playing at eleven in the morning and it was almost 90°. I thought maybe I was getting heat stroke, though I've played harder on hotter days without any trouble. Anyway, we finished the set and I managed to win seven-six in a tie-breaker. Helen's never come within three games of beating me before. She was happy as could be of course, and I didn't say anything because I didn't want to look like a poor loser, but the fact was I was seeing double for almost all the last set. I played the tie-breaker with one eye closed, which helped a little. But I can tell you, I was scared. I didn't know whether I was going blind or what was wrong.

"Well, you know me. I hated to admit it was anything serious so I just went home, took a shower, called the office and told them I wouldn't be in that afternoon, and took a nap. When I woke up I thought I was all right. I didn't seem to be seeing double anymore, but then the evening paper came and when I started to read it, I knew I had been kidding myself. I couldn't read except by closing one eye. And that's the way I've been walking around most of the time for the last two days. I'm amazed Leo didn't notice, but he's been busy with teacher/school-board salary negotiations and hasn't been home much. When I was still having trouble this morning I decided I'd better give up and come in and see you. Your nurse was nice enough to work me into your schedule.''

"Tell me more about this double vision. Is it getting any worse?"

"No," Judy said, "in fact I almost canceled. I think it's a little bit better. But now something new has developed. I'm having trouble walking. Not real bad—most people wouldn't notice it—but I found myself stumbling over nothing several times today. It's as though I lose my balance. Sounds crazy, doesn't it? Maybe it's just my nerves. That's certainly what I hope it is.''

"Have you been having any trouble with your nerves?" I asked.

"Not really," she answered. "You know how I am. I get all worked up whenever I think I'm about to make a big sale. But the real-estate business has been slow lately and there's nothing special bothering me at the office. The kids are fine and even with the school-board negotiations, Leo is his usual easygoing self. I don't really feel nervous. In fact, I don't feel sick at all.''

"Why don't I check you over anyway?" I said. "How long has it been since you've had a complete physical?"

"Two years, I guess," she said. "Fred gave me a good going over before I had Frankie and he was two in June. I suppose I should have been in for a Pap smear, but you know how it is; you keep putting things off.''

"Yes, I know how it is," I said, "I haven't had a complete physical in five years, but don't tell any of my patients that. It would be bad for business. You go on into the examining room and get into one of those gowns. Marge will help you. Then I'm going to give you a thorough going over. Maybe it's all in your head, but we're going to find out.

"And I'm going to have our lab technician get a routine blood and urine test on you. Maybe I'll even get a chest X-ray and an electrocardiogram. Might as well have the works while you're here. Besides, I need the money. Joan needs a new tennis racket."

Judy laughed, went into the examining room, and five minutes later, with my nurse, Marge, in the room, I did a complete physical examination of Judy. All I could find was a difference in the reflexes between her left and right legs; not much, but a definite abnormality. Her electrocardiogram and chest X-ray were both normal, as were her blood and urine analyses. When I finished the examination and the tests were done I told Judy to get dressed.

When she joined me in my office, I could tell from the way she was fidgeting with her handkerchief that she was nervous. I decided to get directly to the point. "Judy," I said, "the only abnormality I can find is in your nervous system. The reflexes in your right leg are much more active than in your left leg. Frankly, I don't know what this means, but it probably means something. I'm no neurologist, as you know, and I think I'd better send you to one. He may want to do some more tests to see if you have some odd neurological disorder."

"Such as?" Judy asked.

"Well," I said, "I don't want to jump to any conclusions but I'm wondering if you might have multiple sclerosis. The double vision, the stumbling, the difference in reflexes all could be signs of that disease. They could also be signs of other diseases and it's still possible they might not mean much, if anything. Anyway, I wouldn't feel safe if we ignored them. I think we ought to try to establish a diagnosis as soon as possible."

"So do I," Judy said. She was on the verge of tears. "You don't really think it's multiple sclerosis, do you, Bill?" she asked. "Don't patients with multiple sclerosis just get more and more paralyzed? If that's true, and I've got the disease, I think I'd really rather be dead." Then she did start to sob.

"Now, Judy," I said, "I know it's difficult to think about things like this and maybe I've mentioned the possibility too soon. But let's get one thing clear; even if you have multiple sclerosis—and I am not saying you do—everyone with the disease doesn't just get progressively paralyzed. A lot of people get completely well for long periods of time and some have only one attack that seems like multiple sclerosis and then never have another. In those patients we never even say they've had multiple sclerosis. Most doctors won't make a definite diagnosis till the patient has had at least two attacks.

"Now, I don't know if you know a neurologist whom you'd like to see. If you do, just give me his name and I'll call him. Otherwise I know a good one in Minneapolis, Dr. Lee Robinson, who I'm sure you'll like. I'll give him a call and make an appointment for you to see him right away; tomorrow if possible. Unless you want to talk to Leo about it first."

"No," Judy said, "I'm sure Leo will agree with me. I can get Helen Fogarty to drive me to Minneapolis tomorrow. Why don't you see if you can set up an appointment."

I called Lee Robinson, told him Judy's story and what I'd found, and he agreed to see her the next day. "Frankly, Bill, just on the strength of what you've told me I think we may as well plan to admit her to the hospital right away. She ought to have an electroencephalogram [brain tracing], a lumbar puncture [to obtain and examine a spinal fluid specimen] and some other tests. No sense in having her make a second trip down. See if she can come and stay for about three days.''

I put my hand over the speaker, told Judy what Lee had said, and she agreed. We then arranged for her to be admitted to Norwood Hospital the next day.

Judy and Lee Robinson got along very well. As I had expected, he did get an electroencephalogram and a spinal fluid examination. Both showed some minor abnormalities but no marked changes. These are findings consistent with multiple sclerosis. There are no tests which absolutely prove the disease exists.

On Friday afternoon Lee discharged Judy and then called me. He told me what he had found. ''I suspect she does have multiple sclerosis, Bill,'' he said, ''but I explained to her that we couldn't yet be certain. We'd have to wait and see how she came along. I told her for now to just lay off the tennis for a couple of weeks, get plenty of rest and eat a balanced diet. I'll see her again in two weeks.''

One week later Judy called me and said, ''Bill, I can hardly believe it—sometimes I think I'm fooling myself—but I'm just about certain I'm getting better. My double vision is completely gone; I can read a book or the paper without any difficulty. And I haven't stumbled or lost my balance for two days. Do you think I could just have had some strange kind of flu?''

''Maybe, Judy,'' I said, ''but it could be that you had an attack of multiple sclerosis and it's going into remission. Remember, I told you that could happen and I'll bet Lee Robinson did too. Now don't get too active. Just take it easy till you see Lee in another week.''

A week later Judy went back to see Robinson. He got another electroencephalogram and did a second spinal tap. He kept her in the hospital overnight and called me when he sent her home the next day. ''All tests are now normal, Bill,'' he said. ''Her reflexes are the same in both legs and both the E.E.G. and spinal fluid are free of any abnormalities. I told her that I can't say she has M.S., nor can I say she hasn't. Time will tell. I told her she could gradually resume her regular activities. Tennis, starting with doubles next week, and half days at her office. Let's hope she doesn't have another attack. She's a very happy woman right now.''

She remained so for the next six months. Then one day she noticed an unusual tingling sensation in the calf of her right leg. The next day the tingling was still there and the double vision was back. She called me and was almost hysterical over the phone.

"Damn," she said. "I'd just about forgotten this stupid disease and now I'm having symptoms again. What do I do now?"

"First, calm down," I said. "You got over your last attack quickly and maybe you'll have the same experience this time. I'd like you to see Lee Robinson again; tomorrow if you can make it. I'm sure he'll work you into his schedule."

"Fine," she said, "I want to know what's going on. I don't care what this is, Bill, I'm going to beat it."

"Great," I said, "That sounds more like the Judy Rankin I know."

The next day, after she'd seen Lee, he called me. "I didn't even bother with anything but a physical and routine lab work, Bill," he said. "Her history is clear and she's got sensory changes in her right leg; she's numb in some places and hypersensitive in others. I'd say there's no doubt she has M.S. I told her to rest again for a couple of weeks and we'd see what happens. I told her this might be her last attack. Let's hope so. She's obviously used to leading a very active life and I'd hate to see her get progressively worse."

When her second attack cleared up, in about three weeks, I asked Judy to come into my office. "Judy," I said, "I'm hopeful, and so is Lee, that you're one of those persons who has a very mild case of multiple sclerosis. Now, if you're sure you really want to know all there is to know about the disease, I'll give you my lecture. It's a mixture of good and bad news. Some patients prefer not knowing what may happen, and that's their privilege.''

"Go on, Bill," she said, "tell me all you know." I was almost certain that's what Judy would say, so I spent the next hour with her talking and answering her questions.

"First," I said, "let me confess that we don't know with certainty what causes multiple sclerosis so we don't have any specific, curative treatment for the disease. We do know that it behaves differently in different people and we treat each case individually. The only warning I'm going to give you is this: stay away from quacks. They love to treat patients with multiple sclerosis because they know, with time, most victims will improve with or without treatment and, whatever the treatment they've used, they'll get credit for what's actually a normal, spontaneous remission. It's difficult to imagine how many multiple sclerosis patients go to quacks out of desperation. I'm sure you won't do that.

"In seventy percent of cases the disease is chronic and relapsing, with both exacerbations and remissions unpredictable in length. Some patients have one or two attacks, then never have a third. In thirty percent of patients the disease never relents and may progress rapidly, causing death in several months or a very few years. Death in multiple sclerosis usually results from repeated infections of either the bladder and kidneys or the lungs, depending on which organs are weakened by the disease. There—now you have the very worst news. But let me assure you again, Judy, both Lee and I think you'll be one of the seventy percent. Now to some medical information.

"Multiple sclerosis is a disease of the nervous system, involving both the brain and the spinal cord and nerves, though the spinal cord and nerves are more often directly affected. The patient develops patchy areas of degeneration of the outer coating of the brain and nerves—called demyelinization—which interferes with transmission of impulses along the nerves to the organs they serve. For example, when the nerves to the bladder become demyelinized, the bladder will not function properly. The patient may not be able to completely empty the bladder and the residual urine becomes an ideal medium for bacteria growth. Similarly, if the nerves to the diaphragm or chest wall muscles are damaged the patient will not breathe deeply, and the chances of developing lung infection increase.

"The incidence of multiple sclerosis is much lower in tropical or near tropical climates than it is in the north; ten cases per hundred thousand population in the south as opposed to sixty cases per hundred thousand in the north.

"The incidence in men is about the same as in women and is the same in whites as in blacks.

"Sixty-seven percent of cases begin between the ages of twenty and forty and ninety-five percent between ten and fifty.

"There is no evidence the disease is hereditary. The theory now most widely accepted is that multiple sclerosis is probably caused by the body's immune reaction to some as yet unidentified virus. This theory is based on the changes in the spinal fluid and by the microscopic examination of tissues removed from multiple sclerosis patients.

"The symptoms of multiple sclerosis, roughly in order of incidence, are weakness; double or blurred vision; loss of coordination; tingling sensations; pain, particularly facial pain; loss of bladder control and dizziness.

"Mental changes may occur, but rarely. It used to be said that euphoria—a feeling of intense happiness—was characteristic of the multiple sclerosis patient. It is probably more accurate to say that the patient is apt to show emotional lability. However, since depression, euphoria and emotional lability are so common in otherwise normal people, mental changes—like so many of the other symptoms—are, even if real, not very helpful in diagnosis.

"The treatment of multiple sclerosis is not uniform. The reason different methods of therapy are chosen by different doctors is that, as I've already emphasized, the course of multiple sclerosis is so unpredictable that it's difficult to determine whether improvement in a particular patient's case is due to the therapy or simply the result of a spontaneous remission.

"Generally, however, for someone who has an acute attack of what appears to be multiple sclerosis, the doctor will hospitalize the patient and use an initial course of cortisone for about three or four weeks. Some doctors will maintain patients on small doses of cortisone or cortisonelike drugs indefinitely, but most physicians feel that such long-term therapy is not only useless but hazardous. Drugs of the cortisone type frequently cause dangerous side effects.

"If the patient suffers from weakness or paralysis of a part of her body, it is important to begin physiotherapy immediately. To neglect the paralyzed limb may lead to contractures and stiffness that will be difficult to reverse. And even though rest is usually recommended for the patient with an acute attack, some physical activity should not only be permitted but encouraged.

"As far as diet is concerned, though many fad diets have been suggested and tried, most physicians agree that any well-balanced diet with an adequate vitamin and mineral content and a caloric intake that maintains ideal weight is all that is necessary. There's no evidence that special diets will slow the progression or delay recurrences of multiple sclerosis.

"I've already mentioned that some patients have one or two attacks of multiple sclerosis and then live a normal life span without any other recurrence.

"Overall, follow-up studies have shown that five

years after the onset of the disease, seventy percent of
patients are still gainfully employed, with occasional
brief interruptions when attacks occur. After ten years,
fifty percent of patients are still working and completely
asymptomatic most of the time. After twenty years,
thirty-five percent of patients are still working and
living near-normal lives. The mortality rate twenty years
after the onset of the disease is only twenty percent—not
much higher than that of the normal population—and
many patients, who first get the disease when relatively
young, will live fifty years or more. Death, as I've mentioned, is usually caused by severe, repeated lung or
bladder infections.

"There were about 500,000 patients with multiple
sclerosis living in the United States in 1979. In all
probability you know one or two patients with the
disease, but may not recognize them as such because
they live perfectly normal lives. I am currently ac-
quainted with four patients who are completely free of
the signs and symptoms of the disease.

"Certainly it is not a pleasant disease to have and, as
I've noted, not all patients manage to lead near-normal
lives. But most do, and with the continuing research
into the cause and treatment, it's probable we'll find a
cure in the near future.

"In the meantime let me repeat; quack practitioners
delight in treating multiple sclerosis patients. Those who
advertise cures—snake venom injections and hyperbaric
oxygen therapy, in which a patient is immersed in a tank
and subjected to very high concentrations of oxygen,
are two current favorites—have as yet no statistical or
experimental proof their therapy can produce any
miraculous cures.

"Now," I said, "you know as much about the disease
as I do, and I may as well confess I've been reading up
on M.S. ever since you first came to see me. Any
questions?"

"None, Bill," she said. "I just want to thank you for

leveling with me. I probably know more about the disease than I need to know, but that's better—at least for me—than not knowing enough. I'm going to try to go on living normally and just pray that I won't have another attack."

It's now more than eight years since Judy's last attack. She has had absolutely no symptoms. Judy had wanted another baby, so in 1973, about a year and a half after her second attack, she got pregnant and now has a second son, Leo Junior. (Most doctors agree that it's perfectly safe for a woman with M.S. to become pregnant but most also believe that she should wait at least a year after she has had an episode of symptoms.)

At forty-one Judy looks as handsome as ever and still plays a very strong game of tennis. She now has her own real estate agency and that, along with her three children, keeps her busy. But she loves life and seems to be enjoying it to the hilt.

One night, when we were at a cocktail party at the golf club, Judy mentioned multiple sclerosis to me. "I know I've been lucky, Bill, and I hope I stay that way. But I think if I do have another attack I'll be able to accept it. I'm the eternal optimist, I guess. I have a feeling I can beat anything or anyone."

I agreed with her. I'm pleased she's done so well and I hope we've seen the last of Judy's M.S. It's another reminder of how little we doctors know about so many different ailments. M.S. may be a rotten disease, but one thing can certainly be said for it. It does—or ought to—keep us doctors humble.

17

The Tumor No One Thought
Would Go Away

Brad Lawrence is 6 feet tall and weighed 170 pounds when he was sixteen years old, in February 1970. He is a friend of my eldest son, and a frequent visitor to our house. Since we have six children, an old Brunswick pool table that can be converted to a Ping-Pong table simply by putting the wooden top on it, and a hi-fi set in the basement, our home has been a natural gathering place for kids as they've gradually progressed through high school. (Our children are Jim, twenty-five; Jody, twenty-four; Billy, twenty-three; Annie, twenty-one, Julius, nineteen; and Mary, seventeen—their ages as of 1980.)

Brad's father and mother are pleasant, quiet people. Joan and I don't see them socially since they don't go out often. Brad's father, Dick, runs a small farm. He owns only forty acres but he farms another 240, dividing the profit—if any—with the owner. This, incidentally, is very common practice in our area. Unless a farmer inherits land, it's difficult to earn enough money farming to buy it. Some farmers have done it, but not many.

About three o'clock on a Wednesday afternoon, Brad's mother, Georgette, brought him to my office.

"I'm surprised to see you here, Brad," I said. "You didn't look very sick to me when I saw you at my house a few days ago." Brad just smiled; he's a quiet, bashful sort of boy.

"He isn't really sick," his mother said. "In fact, he didn't want to come in to see you, but I insisted. He has some sort of lump in his neck. He had a sore throat about two months ago and that's when we first noticed it. I thought maybe the lump would go away when his sore throat got better but it hasn't. In fact, if anything, it's bigger. Dick and I thought we'd better have you check it."

I did, and the lump was easily felt. It seemed to be about the size of a golf ball. It was firm and located about two inches below the right angle of his jaw, in front of the muscle that runs from the jaw to the breast bone. I looked in his mouth, which was perfectly normal, then did a complete physical examination which disclosed no other abnormalities. I had our technician examine a blood smear and do a urinalysis, both of which were normal.

When I'd finished my examination I told Mrs. Lawrence that the lump was the only abnormality I could find. "To be perfectly honest," I said, "I don't know what it is. These neck lumps are often a puzzle. It's possible that what I'm feeling is just a bunch of inflamed glands—lymph nodes—that got infected when Brad had the sore throat. However, that's just a guess and I really don't think that's what it is. To get a lump that size from infection would be extremely unusual.

"It could be some sort of congenital cyst. When the embryo develops it goes through a stage when there are gill-like structures in the neck; sometimes these linger on as cysts. Usually, however, they get infected and swell up long before the child reaches sixteen. What it all boils down to is that Brad has a lump in his neck that doesn't belong there and even though it doesn't hurt him or make him sick, I think it ought to come out. In all probability it's nothing serious, but I think we'd better make certain.''

"Could it be a tumor?" Mrs. Lawrence asked.

"It could be," I admitted. "In fact, technically it is a tumor because all 'tumor' means is 'a swelling' and it's certainly that. But if you mean could it be a malignant tumor—a cancer of some sort—I have to say yes. I think that's unlikely but, since I can't say positively that it's not, we ought to get it out. I wouldn't want to take even a small chance of leaving a malignant tumor in Brad. Even if it's benign it shouldn't be there and if it's getting bigger, as you seem to think it is, then that's all the more reason to remove it soon. The smaller it is, the easier it should be to take out.

"I know you'll want to talk it over with Dick, but try to make up your mind as soon as you can. Just call me and I can put Brad on the operating schedule at your convenience. However, I'd prefer to do it on a Tuesday or Friday when our pathologist is here. Then he can examine the lump under the microscope immediately and give us an answer. The operation I do may depend on what sort of tumor it is. And, unless I find a bigger problem than I expect, I should think Brad could go home a day or two after the operation. We'll take his stitches out here in the office.''

Mrs. Lawrence called me at home that night. "Dick and Brad and I talked it over at supper," she said. "We all agreed we'd like to get it over with. Can you do it Friday?''

"Sure," I said, "just get Brad into the hospital at about 7:00 P.M. on Thursday. I have a gallbladder operation to do Friday morning, but I think I'll switch cases around and do Brad first. The pathologist will be there and you won't be in suspense as long as you might be otherwise. My gallbladder patient won't mind.''

One of the nice things about practicing in a small town is that you can make a switch like this without difficulty. In a big hospital, with a lot of surgeons on staff, it's often difficult to make last-minute changes. Most surgeons prefer the first operating hours not only because they are freshest then but because it enables them to plan their day. If they have the third or fourth case on the schedule, they can only make a rough estimate of how long the earlier cases will take and sometimes they can be off by several hours.

Friday morning, I operated on Brad. Like most teenagers he wasn't awfully concerned about what I might find—not nearly so much as his parents or I were. Young people rarely think about dying. I'm sure Brad didn't dwell for more than a few seconds on the possibility that this lump in his neck might be a cancer. He felt too well.

To my chagrin, when I'd made the incision through the skin and superficial fat and pulled the muscle out of the way to expose the lump, I found it was stuck very firmly to the deep structures in the neck; the blood vessels to and from the brain and the nerves that run to the vocal cords and tongue. I tried very carefully to free it up, but it was so adherent to the major arteries and veins that I was reluctant to try and peel it off. I don't do any elective blood vessel surgery—just emergency cases in which a delay in treatment means the loss of a limb and/or a life—and though we keep a few synthetic blood vessels in our hospital, I rarely use them. In this case I was also dealing with a blood vessel that supplied a major portion of the blood to the brain and, if I broke into it so that I would have to clamp it off even for a few minutes, it was highly probable Brad's brain would be severely damaged.

I decided that "discretion was the better part of valor" and didn't attempt to remove the entire mass. Instead, I took three small pieces from different areas of the tumor so that our pathologist could study them under the microscope and tell me whether these were just inflamed glands or, as I now suspected, a malignancy of some sort.

While our pathologist was doing a "frozen section" on one part of one piece, I closed the wound. No matter what the diagnosis I had no intention of doing any more operating on this growth. If it was the sort of tumor that responded to radiation treatment I'd refer him to a radiologist; if it was the kind of growth best treated by surgical removal, I'd refer him to a friend of mine in Minneapolis who did a lot of blood vessel surgery; and, of course, it was still possible that these were simply inflamed glands which would shrivel up as the inflammation subsided, perhaps after antibiotic treatment.

It took me about ten minutes to close the incision, by which time Dr. Bob Fedor, our pathologist, had had a chance to study the section under the microscope. "What's the answer, Bob?" I asked.

"Darned if I know, Bill," he said. "It's a strange-looking devil. It might be a lymphosarcoma but if it is, it's an odd-looking one. I'm reluctant to give you an answer till I have a chance to study the permanent sections." Bob Fedor is an excellent pathologist; one of the kind who, wisely, isn't afraid to say, "I don't know" when, rarely, that's the case.

"Fine," I said, "just give me a call when you've got an answer."

"Should know by Monday," he said. "I'll call your office."

I went out and explained to the Lawrences what I'd found and done. "I hate to keep you in suspense," I said, "but we'll have to wait till Monday. I'll let Brad go home tomorrow and if you call me late on Monday afternoon I'll let you know what has to be done."

The Lawrences accepted the news graciously and promised to call me Monday. When they did I had to stall them again. "I'm sorry," I said, "but Dr. Fedor still isn't sure what the tumor is. It's an odd one. He's going to have some other pathologists look at it. Call me again on Thursday." It is only sensible for a pathologist to ask other pathologists to give an opinion as to diagnosis when the tumor is an unusual one.

By Thursday, Bob had reports from three other pathologists, including a professor of pathology at the University of Minnesota. The consensus was that this was a chemodectoma (also called a nonchromaffin paraganglioma), a very rare tumor that sometimes begins in a tiny (about 1/8-inch in diameter) white structure called the carotid body that normally lies behind the major carotid arteries to the neck. The carotid body helps to regulate the carbon dioxide level of the blood.

I asked Mr. and Mrs. Lawrence to come to my office on Thursday so I could explain the problem to them. I find that showing illustrations—either sketches that I make or illustrations from a surgical text—often helps the patient or relatives understand the problem. When I'd finished my explanation I said, "Usually this is a benign tumor, but once in a while we run across one that grows rapidly and has some malignant cells in it. In either case the only reasonable treatment is removal. If you agree, I'm going to refer Brad to a surgeon in Minneapolis who does a lot of surgery on the blood vessels of the neck. To be perfectly honest, I don't think I should do the operation. I might get away with it, but the doctor to whom I'm going to refer you has much more experience with this sort of problem than I do. If Brad were my son, this is the man to whom I'd send him." (That's a rule I often apply to unusual cases; if the patient was a member of my family, where or by whom would I want to have him or her treated? That's where I send the patient.)

Brad's folks agreed with my decision and I referred him to a surgeon I'll call John Barrett. After doing additional studies, including special X-rays of the neck arteries which showed that the tumor hadn't invaded the vessels, John operated on Brad two weeks after I had operated on him. He called me immediately afterward.

(We already had a microscopic diagnosis of the portion I had removed. Now the pathologist would have to take multiple sections through the mass that John had removed and then do a prolonged, detailed examination to see if there were any malignant cells in the specimen. This sort of study cannot be adequately done with frozen sections; nor, since the operation was completed, was there any need for an immediate answer.)

"Bill," he said, "that was one hell of a tumor. Assuming it is a chemodectoma, it's the biggest one anyone on the hospital staff has ever seen. I did my best to get it all out but it was so adherent to the carotid arteries and the jugular vein that I'm sure I left some bits behind. We'll just have to hope it's benign; if it is, maybe he'll be all right. But if it's malignant, then I'm afraid he isn't cured. Sorry, I did all I reasonably could do."

"I'm sure of that, John," I said. "I knew it was going to be a darn tough job. Have you spoken to the Lawrences?"

"Yes, just a few minutes ago. I told them just what I've told you. Incidentally, I'm afraid I may have cut the recurrent laryngeal nerve on the right [the nerve to the right vocal cord]. It ran right through the tumor and there wasn't any way I could spare it. I've warned his parents that Brad may be hoarse for a while. They understand."

"Let's hope it's benign," I said. "Call me when you have all the pathology reports."

"Don't worry," John said. "I'll let you know."

A week later, after several pathologists had again examined the new microscopic slides, John phoned me. "It looks bad," he said, "It's a chemodectoma—all the pathologists agree on that—but there are several areas in the tumor where the cells are very wild. I'm afraid he's in trouble.

"I've talked the case over with our radiologist. He says they could radiate him now in the hope of knocking off any remaining cells, but since these tumors are relatively radio-resistant he thinks we may as well wait and see if it recurs. In the meantime Brad has been recovering nicely and he's ready to go home. He'll be in to see you in a week so you can check his incision. I'll see him again in six months."

"Damn," I said, "I was hoping it would be benign. I guess we'll just have to hope that anything you left behind is slow-growing. We'll see."

For the first year there was no sign of a recurrence. Brad's hoarseness improved gradually and he continued to lead an active life. Then, after eighteen months, his mother noticed a lump in the upper end of the incision. It was about the size of a marble and there was little doubt in my mind that it was recurrent tumor. I sent Brad back to John, who reoperated, found the tumor was stuck to the base of the skull and not removable, took a biopsy, which confirmed the diagnosis, and closed up.

"May as well send him to the radiologist," John said. "It could be one of the rare ones that responds to radiation. There's nothing else to do anyway and I hate to just let the poor kid go. The radiation shouldn't make him sick, so it's probably worth doing." I agreed, as did Brad's family.

The radiologist, an expert in tumor treatment, wasn't optimistic either but he agreed to give it a try. Over the next five weeks he administered twenty-eight cobalt treatments, shooting the X-rays in through several different "portals" so as to do as little damage as possible to the skin. Even so, Brad got a fairly severe radiation burn which responded to a cortisone cream. "Now we just wait and see," I told Brad's folks, "and pray, if you're so inclined. There's nothing more to be done."

The tumor responded beautifully to the radiation. Within two weeks of the end of treatment it had shriveled away so we couldn't even feel it. But we had more or less expected that. What concerned us was the possibility—the probability—that a few cells would survive the X-ray bombardment and would start to regrow in a few months.

Well, as you've probably guessed since this is a book of hope, it is now seven years since the radiation treatment ended and there is no sign of a recurrence. Brad, who is now twenty-five, is married and has a child. He is a big, strong, healthy young man. There is no doubt in my mind—nor in the minds of any of the others who helped treat him—that Brad is cured. Had he been going to have a recurrence, he would almost certainly have had it within two years and definitely within five. His life expectancy is now normal—as even the company which recently sold him life insurance realizes.

Brad's story, not to belabor what I hope is a reasonably obvious point, demonstrates that although there are times when a patient should be allowed to die comfortably—without, for example, undergoing radiation in a futile attempt to "cure" a tumor known to be resistant to radiation, particularly when the radiation may cause nausea or painful skin burns—the decision to forego that treatment should not be made when there is even a minimal hope that a cure, or even a substantial increase in longevity, can be obtained. It should particularly not be made when the patient is young, otherwise healthy, with a long life expectancy. And the patient and the family should join in the decision making.

Before I recommended that we go ahead with the radiation I had a long talk with Brad's parents. I made it clear that we could promise nothing, that we were suggesting radiation treatment simply because there was no other reasonable alternative, and that, even though we expected some skin reaction, we didn't think it would cause so much pain as to make the radiation treatment unreasonable. I emphasized the positive when I talked to Brad, who was then only eighteen, but I made certain his parents knew the chance of a cure was a long shot. To raise unreasonable expectations would not have been fair.

The second, and I hope obvious point is that when a physician encounters a disease he has rarely seen before, he has a moral obligation to seek the help and advice of others more experienced. I'd never seen a chemodectoma before; neither, for that matter, had John Barrett. But John had had considerably more experience with the type of surgery required in Brad's case, so he was a logical choice to do the operation.

And I'm delighted that the case has had such a happy ending.

18

Life's Less of a Gamble if
You Use Your Head

      Betty Ramier was thirty-six in 1970 when she came to our clinic for her annual physical examination. At that time Betty, who had married at thirty, had two children, a daughter, Sandy, two, and a son, Jerry, four. She had been taking birth control pills for the two years since the birth of her son.

After I'd completed my examination, which included a pelvic examination and Pap smear, I told her, "Everything seems fine, Betty. We'll have to wait a few days before the result of the Pap smear is back, but your heart, lungs, blood pressure and everything else are normal. Your uterus feels normal and the cervix [the neck of the uterus, which can be seen when we do a vaginal examination] looks just as it should. Call me in a week if I haven't phoned you with the results of the Pap smear; sometimes I forget to call patients."

"I won't forget, Dr. Nolen," she said. "And, by the way, I'm going to quit taking those birth control pills after my next menstrual period, which is due in two weeks. George and I have decided we'd really like to have another child."

"Fine," I said. "Joan and I have six children, as you know, but we started back in the days when big families

176

were more popular than they are now. They're awfully expensive to raise, I can assure you, but we've never regretted having them." Betty left and I went in to see my next patient.

Five days later the report on Betty's Pap smear came back. The pathologist wrote that he saw some "suspicious" cells; they weren't definitely malignant, but neither were they quite normal. The report made me uneasy.

Before I go any further I'd better explain what a Pap smear is. The name comes from Dr. George Papanicolaou who, in 1941, devised a test which enables us to make an early diagnosis of cancer of the cervix, the portion of the uterus where most cancers begin. In a Pap test the doctor, while doing a vaginal examination, uses a disposable wooden spatula to scrape a few cells from the mouth of the cervix. The procedure is painless. The cells are then placed on a glass slide, covered with a preservative, and sent to the pathologist. He uses special dyes to stain the cells, then examines them to see if there are any abnormalities of cell structure which suggest early cancer or other diseases. The test has now been done for so many years that preliminary screening of the slides can be safely done by technicians trained to identify any abnormalities.

After the report had been placed on my desk, I called Betty. "Betty," I said, "I hate to tell you this, and please try not to be too alarmed, but the Pap smear I did last week showed some cells that looked suspicious. They aren't definitely cancer cells, but they aren't quite normal either. The pathologist suggests we repeat the test in three months, but I know you want to get pregnant again if you can, so I'd suggest that we admit you to the hospital now so that I can take a cone of tissue out. That way, we can get a definite answer immediately."

"I'm all for it, Dr. Nolen," Betty said. "Even if I didn't want to get pregnant I'd hate to wait around for three months wondering if I had cancer.'' That was the reaction I'd expected from Betty; in fact, it's the reaction I get from most women. Understandably, they hate the suspense of not knowing whether they have a life-threatening disease; though a three month delay after a suspicious Pap test (Class II, benign with some atypical cells), even if the later test is read as Class IV (some atypical cells, but not conclusive for cancer) would probably not decrease Betty's chances of being cured.

Three days later Betty was admitted to the hospital and, under a light general anesthetic, I removed a cone of tissue from the cervix. The cervical mouth is more or less round and a cone of tissue is a circular sampling of the entire mouth of the cervix. It goes deeper than the Pap test, which yields only the most superficial cells, and it produces tissue from the entire circumference of the cervix. Betty was up and around in the afternoon after the operation and I let her go home that night.

Another few days passed, with both of us in suspense, and then we got the pathologist's report. He had spotted a few superficial cells which he felt obliged to classify as "atypical," but there was no evidence of cancer. He felt we had probably removed all the potentially dangerous cells.

I explained the report to Betty. "There were a few suspicious changes within the cells, but no spread outside those few superficial cells and no malignant cells. Now we have to make a decision. We can leave your uterus in, I can do a repeat Pap smear in three months, and then, if it's negative and you still want to get pregnant, I think it will be safe to go ahead. Or, if you decide you don't want to run even that small risk, we can remove your uterus now."

"Let me talk it over with George tonight, Dr. Nolen," Betty said. "I'll call you tomorrow."

"Fine," I said, "personally, I think either course is very safe."

When Betty called me the next day she said, "We've

decided we'd still like to have another child. I'll stay off the Pill but we'll use another form of birth control for three months. Then, if everything is O.K., I'll get pregnant."

"Be sure to let me know if you do any spotting between periods, won't you?" I said.

"Don't worry," Betty replied, "I have to confess I'm going to be a little nervous till this is all over."

Betty Ramier had always been a self-confident woman. She had graduated from the University of Colorado in 1955. Her major was in history and she had decided to go on and get a master's degree at the University of Wisconsin. She held part-time jobs most of the time and was repeatedly granted scholarships. After completing her master's, she accepted a teaching job at a junior college near Minneapolis and continued her studies, earning a doctorate in history. Her father was a farmer who barely earned enough to support his family, so Betty had been forced to do all this on her own. She had met George, her husband, while they were both students at Colorado. After they had married, George, an engineer, was offered a position with a small manufacturing firm in Litchfield and Betty got a job teaching history in a nearby town. Betty and George had moved to Litchfield in 1961, a year after Joan and I had moved here, and we'd become reasonably close friends, playing bridge and going to Minneapolis to the theater with them occasionally.

Knowing Betty and George well, I wasn't surprised when they reacted as they did to the news I had given them. I know other women who I am certain would have given up the idea of having another child and asked for an immediate hysterectomy instead. What was to Betty an acceptable risk would not necessarily have been acceptable to someone else.

Three months later I repeated the Pap test. This time the report was, "Normal cells." Betty was pregnant two months later and had a second healthy son, Ralph, nine months after that. After this birth Betty said, "I couldn't be happier. I'm so glad we decided to go ahead. But I have to admit, this is it. Three are going to be enough."

For the next three years I did Pap smears on Betty every six months; she was using an intrauterine coil for birth control. Finally, in 1977, a smear again revealed abnormal cells. This time the report read, "Probably very early malignant change," and there was no hesitation on Betty, George's or my part. I performed a hysterectomy from which she made an uneventful recovery. When the pathologist examined the uterus he found only a few, very early malignant cells, confined to the neck of the cervix.

It's three years since her operation, Betty is doing very nicely and I'm sure she's cured. In fact, I was virtually certain I'd cured her on the day I performed the hysterectomy. The cure rate of cervical cancer, detected on a routine Pap smear, ought to be almost one hundred percent.

I've written about Betty's case not because it suggests anything particular about a patient's will to live—though Betty has always been a vigorous, courageous person—but because it demonstrates how one person, using the mind God gave him, was able to devise a simple, painless test that has, over the last fifty years, helped reduce the mortality rate from cancer of the uterus from twenty-eight per hundred thousand to seven per hundred thousand; and of those who still die annually of cancer of the cervix, almost all are patients who have neglected to take advantage of this remarkable test. They wait till they have abnormal bleeding or pelvic pain or some other symptom before they come to see their doctor, at which time, if the symptom is due to cancer, the cancer may well have grown beyond the point where it can be cured by surgery, radiation, drugs or any combination thereof.

We can spend all the money we want on "basic"

research. We can make available every possible test, pill or operation that scientists devise. But unless patients take advantage of these things, unless they go to their doctors when they develop signs or symptoms that suggest disease, it will all be in vain.

Betty's case had a happy outcome because she was smart enough to take care of herself. In the final analysis, that's what we must all do.

19

Living Long—
and Comfortably—with Cancer

People often seem to think, and act, as if all types of cancer were the same. They aren't, of course. For example, the most common form is skin cancer. There are an estimated 300,000 new cases of skin cancer every year. Yet, in twenty years of practice I've only known of one patient who died of the ordinary forms of skin cancer (I'm excluding malignant melanoma, a relatively rare form of the disease, which is often lethal). That patient simply refused all treatment until the cancer finally grew so large it couldn't be removed. But under all reasonable circumstances the ordinary forms of skin cancer—the kind, for example, that you get from exposure to too much sun—can be easily treated. (I am not suggesting that you go out and broil in the sun all year, particularly if you have developed one skin cancer. I am saying that, even if you do, you can easily be cured by excision of the growth.) The American Cancer Society doesn't even bother to report the incidence of deaths from ordinary skin cancer (basal cell or epidermoid) because the incidence is so low.

There's another relatively common form of cancer, however, that annually causes about ten percent of all cancer deaths in males, but with which a patient can live comfortably for many years. (When I say that it causes ten percent of all cancer deaths in males, the reader should realize that this represents only fifteen deaths per 100,000 population, and these deaths occur, ordinarily, in very elderly men.) I am writing, if you haven't guessed, about cancer of the prostate. I write about it to try and relieve the terror of those who may have the disease or know someone who does.

Bert Everson, a farmer who lives a few miles from Litchfield, is an excellent example not only of the way patients react to the diagnosis of cancer but of the way prostatic cancer commonly behaves.

Bert first came to see me in 1964, when he was sixty-four years old. "I'm not really sick, Doc," he said, "it's just that I can't get a decent night's sleep anymore. I wake up about three times every night because I have to piss. It's annoying."

"Have you tried not drinking any liquids after supper, Bert?" I asked.

"Yes, I tried that," he said, "In fact, all I have with supper is one cup of coffee; I used to have two or three. And I take a leak before I go to bed. Doesn't do any good. Two hours later, I'm up again. Can't you give me a pill or something to help me sleep?"

"Not so fast, Bert," I said, "let me examine you first."

When I did I found nothing wrong—Bert has always been a hard worker and is a big muscular man—until I did a rectal examination. The prostate gland, which surrounds the urethra (the lower opening of the urinary bladder), can be felt by pressing on the front wall of the rectum. Bert's prostate was about twice normal size. Not only that, but it was hard and irregular. It's fairly easy to tell, simply by feeling the prostate through the rectal wall, whether it has cancer in it. I was reasonably certain Bert's did.

When I finished the rectal examination, during which Bert constantly but good-naturedly complained, I asked

him to empty his bladder and give us a urine sample. I
then told him I now wanted to check and see how much
urine was left in his bladder.

"How you gonna do that, Doc?" he asked.

"I'm going to ask you to slip down your pants, lie
down on my examining table, and then I'm going to
pass a narrow rubber tube called a catheter up your
penis into your bladder and drain off whatever urine
you didn't get rid of."

"Damn it, Doc," he said, "that sounds like it'll
hurt."

"Come on, Bert," I said, "you're supposed to be a
big tough guy. Honestly, it will be a little bit uncomfortable but not bad."

"Oh, all right," he said, "I suppose you've got to
have your way." Reluctantly he did as I asked and I
drained two and a half ounces of urine from his bladder, which I showed him.

"What's that mean?" he asked.

"It means," I said, "that when you think you're
emptying your bladder, you aren't. You're leaving
behind two and a half ounces. That means that when
your kidneys make more urine while you're sleeping, it
doesn't take long before your bladder is full and you get
the urge to void. That's why you wake up so often
during the night.

"The reason you can't empty your bladder, Bert, is
that your prostate gland is enlarged; I can feel it when I
examine your rectum. The prostate blocks the opening
of your bladder."

"What can you do about that, Doc?" he asked.

"I can't do anything, Bert, because I don't do
prostate surgery anymore. But I can get a urologist—a
doctor who specializes in surgery of the kidneys and
prostate—to come out here and open up a bigger
passage in that prostate of yours. We give you an
anesthetic and then he passes a metal tube in through
the opening of your penis and he cuts out the parts of

the prostate that are blocking the opening. He leaves one of these catheters in for a few days and then you can go home.''

"Doesn't sound too bad.''

"No, it doesn't and it isn't, Bert. But I have to tell you one other thing. From the way your prostate feels I suspect it's enlarged because there's cancer in it. After your operation, if the pathologist tells us it is a cancer, then we'll probably suggest that you have your testicles removed because the male hormone they produce may make prostatic cancer grow and spread. I have to tell you too, Bert, that removing your testicles will make you impotent.''

Bert had been sitting on one of the chairs in my examination room but now he got up and picked up his cap and jacket. "You just lost me, Doc,'' he said, "I'm going to go right on getting up every couple of hours. If I've got a cancer I'm just going to keep going till it kills me. There's no way you're going to chop me up. I know damn well that when you've got cancer, that's it.''

"Now listen, Bert,'' I said, "You know me well enough to be confident I'm not going to feed you any nonsense. There are cancers and there are cancers. I'm not saying we're going to cure you, to even have a chance at that we'd have to take out your whole prostate and that's a big operation that might cause you more troubles so later you'd need to use a catheter all the time. What I'm telling you is we can do a relatively simple operation, have you out of the hospital in five days, and in all probability keep you alive and well for another ten or twenty years, when you'd probably die of pure cantankerousness anyway. Come on now. Be reasonable. Even if it's cancer, if you don't want your testicles out, we'll leave them; but we'll at least have to put you on a female hormone so the cancer won't come back.''

"Not for me, Doc,'' he said. "Thanks but no thanks. I know enough about cancer to know you can't beat it.

I'm going to enjoy whatever time I have left.''

"Bert," I said, "I can't make you have this operation against your will, but I've leveled with you. Now, if you go home that damn prostate's just going to get bigger and bigger till you won't be able to go at all.''

"I'll take my chances, Doc," Bert said. Then he stuck out his hand. "No hard feelings, I hope,'' he said as we shook.

"None, Bert," I answered. "Call me if you change your mind.'' Bert is a stubborn devil and I knew there was no sense arguing with him. I'd give him two months and then if he hadn't called, I'd call him.

Six weeks later he phoned me. "Goddammit, Doc, it looks as if you're right. It's getting so I can hardly piss at all anymore. I guess I'm going to have to have that reaming. When can you set it up?''

I looked at the operating schedule. "How about next week, Bert?" I asked. "You come in on Sunday night so I can get some blood tests and kidney X-rays. The urologist will be here on Wednesday.''

"All right," he said, "but one other thing. You leave my balls right where they are.''

"OK, Bert," I said. "Whatever you say.'' We wouldn't have done an orchiectomy (removal of the testicles) till we had the pathology report back anyway. Time enough to discuss that later.

Bert sailed through the operation. The urologist cut out a big segment of the prostate that was blocking the lower end of the bladder and five days later Bert was home. Some patients who have had prostatic surgery need a couple of weeks before they have full control of their voiding mechanism, but Bert never had any problems. When I saw him in my office two weeks later he was delighted. "I've slept seven hours straight every night for the last two weeks," he said. "I feel like a new man.''

"Great, Bert," I said. "I'm pleased. Unfortunately, I have to tell you that, as we suspected, it was a cancer.

Now I know how you feel about having your testicles removed, so I'm not going to push you on that, but I think you ought to go on stilbestrol, a female hormone. If you don't, then that cancer is going to start growing again and you'll plug up. And it's possible it might spread somewhere else in your body; usually when it spreads it goes to the spine.''

"Goddammit, Doc, what will those female hormones do to my sex life?''

"I'm afraid they'll end it, Bert," I said. "Just having your prostate reamed won't make you impotent, though it often changes things so that the sperm shoots back into the bladder rather than out through the penis. But if we put you on the female hormones, you'll be impotent.''

"Well, Doc," Bert said, "I'll be honest with you. I haven't been the greatest stud in the world for the last couple of years anyway. I've already talked it over with my wife and she says she'd rather have me alive, well and unable to get it up than dead with a hard-on. I guess I'll take the pills.''

"Your wife's a smart woman, Bert," I said. "But of course I've known that ever since I met her. When was it—two years ago—that I took her gallbladder out?''

"Three years ago," Bert said. "And she's been fine since. She trusts you.''

"That's nice to hear, Bert," I said.

Bert started on one stilbestrol tablet a day in 1964. Eight years later, despite the stilbestrol, he had to have a second transurethral resection (the fancy name for a T.U.R. or a reaming of the prostate) because of increased difficulty voiding. Now, in 1980, sixteen years since his cancer was diagnosed, Bert is still hale and hearty, helping his sons on the farm. He's eighty years old and has lived sixteen years with his prostatic cancer; it's still there and it doesn't bother him a bit.

I shouldn't leave the impression that this is the only way to treat cancer of the prostate; it isn't. In young patients, with small tumors, some urologists will do what is called a radical perineal prostatectomy, which may result in a complete removal of the prostate and a cure of the disease. It also often results in impotency, sterility and, frequently, incontinence. It isn't an operation that is widely done.

In the last few years there have also been reports from some centers which suggest that giving female hormones to patients with cancer of the prostate, while they admittedly protect the patient from his cancer, may cause premature death from heart disease. Supposedly the stilbestrol causes arteriosclerosis to develop more quickly than it otherwise might in the arteries to the heart.

This may or may not be true. What is certainly true is that the vast majority of patients with cancer of the prostate—eighty to ninety percent I'd guess (the figures aren't reported or available)—are treated as we treated Bert Everson, and that most live comfortably with their cancer for many years. We also know that if a thorough microscopic examination of the prostate is done on every man who dies of an unrelated disease, in fourteen percent of men over fifty cancer will be found and that in most of these patients (65.8 percent) the cancer will not have produced any symptoms or even have been detected during the patient's life.

Bert Everson is an excellent example of the fact that you can live long and comfortably with cancer.

20

Out of a Wheelchair, On to the Golf Course

Louise Daly was fifty-three in 1968 when she first began to have trouble with her knees. "It's the same every morning, Dr. Nolen," she told me. "When I wake up, my knees are so stiff it's all I can do to bend them enough to get my stockings on. After I've been up for an hour or so, they loosen up, but by the end of the day they're always sore and usually the right one is swollen. I go home and put a heating pad on them and it helps; the soreness goes away. But I still find myself limping around in the evening. Tom and I used to enjoy going dancing on Saturday nights but now that's out of the question. I've tried it once or twice but the next day my knees are so painful I can barely make it out of bed. Isn't there something you can do to help? I shouldn't be crippled like this at my age."

I'd known Louise almost since I'd moved to Litchfield. She worked as a teller in a local bank. I knew she wasn't a complainer; I'd seen her through several severe gallbladder attacks before I'd finally convinced her to let me take her gallbladder out in 1965. She could tolerate pain as well as the average person. If she said her knees were hurting I could be sure she wasn't exaggerating.

Louise hadn't had any significant knee trouble till after I had removed her gallbladder. I always warn patients with gallstones, who had been having severe gallbladder attacks after dietary indiscretion, that they'll have to be very careful after I've removed their gallbladders. Otherwise, once they find they can eat whatever they want without worrying about pain, they are likely to eat more than they need and put on weight. This had happened to Louise. She had been a stocky woman when I operated on her—about 5'8" and 155 pounds—but in the three years since her operation, despite repeated warnings from me and several brief and unsuccessful attempts at dieting, she had blossomed to 180 pounds. She'd had occasional arthritis pain in her knees for years but it hadn't been till she gained the extra twenty-five pounds that the pain and stiffness became so severe.

"Louise," I said, "how many times have I told you that if you'd lose weight your arthritis wouldn't be so bad?"

"I know, I know," she said, "and I've tried. Honestly, it just seems to me that if I eat anything at all I gain weight. I'm hardly eating now and I can't lose an ounce. Are you sure I don't need some thyroid pills?"

I don't know how often I've heard that question. The figure is in the high hundreds at least. Almost nobody will admit that overeating is the cause of their weight gain. Invariably they'll want to blame their thyroid gland or some other metabolic defect as the cause of their obesity. Yet in fewer than one patient in a thousand is "low thyroid" or any other metabolic disease the cause of their trouble. It's simply too many calories coming in and too few being burned up. Years ago I got tired of arguing that point. Now, if the patient requests it, I'll do blood studies to check their thyroid function. Only then will they really believe me. (Admittedly, this is one small example of the sort of "prophylactic" medicine that contributes to rising medical expenses, but with obese patients it's almost a necessity if I'm to have any success at all in persuading them to diet.)

"How long has it been since we X-rayed your knees?" I asked.

"About two years, I think, Dr. Nolen."

I checked her record and found she was right. So, after examining her—the right knee was slightly swollen and there was some limitation of motion in both knees—I ordered repeated X-rays. I wanted to see if there were more arthritic changes now than there had been two years earlier.

There were. It's not unusual to find some evidence of arthritis in the knees. In patients over forty, X-rays of the spine and knees may reveal at least minor arthritic changes even if the patient has no symptoms; these are the "wear and tear" changes of osteoarthritis, the result of years of pounding on these joints.

The arthritis in Louise's knee joints was, however, considerably more than would ordinarily be expected. She had bone spurs jutting out from the margins of the joints and there were rough spots on the bone ends where particles of bone or cartilage had presumably broken off, the typical changes of osteoarthritis, only more severe than in the average person. There were enough changes in Louise's joints to explain her symptoms.

I showed Louise the films we had just taken and let her compare them with the earlier X-rays. "You can see for yourself, Louise," I said, pointing out the changes, "there's much more joint damage now than there was two years ago. Things are getting worse. Now we have to decide what to do about it."

"There has to be something you can do," Louise said, "I just can't go on like this. I'd quit work if I could, but we need the money. We've still got two children in high school and Tom doesn't earn enough for us. We could get by, I suppose, but it would be tough." Tom worked as a janitor for several small businesses in town. He was a heavy drinker, as I and everyone else in town knew, and I'm sure Louise wasn't exaggerating when she said she needed her job.

"There are a lot of things we can do, Louise, but let's start with the basics; first, you absolutely must lose weight. If you don't, everything else will be in vain. Even if we have to progress to surgery—which I don't think is either necessary or wise right now—the operations will be more effective if you're lighter when they're done. I'm going to put you on a thousand-calorie diet and I want you to stick with it. Every week you stop in here and we'll have one of the nurses weigh you. That's the only way I can be certain that you're sincerely trying.

"Now, let me explain something. There are no 'magic' diets, despite all the nonsense that gets published in books and magazines. There's just one formula on which weight control is based and that is that the calories you take in have to be fewer than the calories you burn up in the same period. If that's true, you'll lose weight; if it isn't, you'll gain weight. We have a simple thousand-calorie diet sheet that we'll give you along with a little handbook that gives the caloric value of most foods, so you can substitute if you wish. That's all you need as a diet guide; don't waste your money on any of these fad diet books. They won't do anything for you that these simple caloric sheets can't do.

"I don't want to frighten you, Louise, but we've reached a critical point. Either you lose weight or, despite anything I or anyone else can do, you may find yourself unable to walk." I could see that I'd frightened Louise, but I was being honest and it seemed to me as if fear might be a necessary motivating factor. It often is where weight loss is concerned.

In any case, it worked. Six months later, after losing fifteen pounds, Louise's symptoms were much less severe. I had prescribed the usual arthritis treatment—two aspirin every four hours and heat to the knees a couple of times a day—but I had had her on that regimen before. The weight loss made the difference.

"I'm much better, Dr. Nolen," she said. "We even went dancing last Saturday. I was fairly stiff Sunday but not nearly as bad as I used to be."

"Great, Louise," I said. "Now don't slip back."

"Don't worry," she said, "I'm so happy to be better you couldn't force a piece of cake down me and everyone tells me I look a lot better too. I'm going to try and lose another ten pounds."

Louise did and for two years her arthritis was much better. Then, despite the fact that she had maintained her weight loss—a feat only achieved by about ten percent of those who initially lose weight; at least ninety percent of those who diet to lose weight will have gained it all back, usually with a few extra pounds, within eighteen months of their ''successful'' dieting—Louise began to have more knee trouble. The arthritic changes had progressed, as our newest X-rays showed, and even with her reduced weight Louise was becoming more and more crippled. I tried cortisone injections into the knees, with some transient benefit, and finally put her on oral cortisone, which she didn't tolerate very well. She developed a small duodenal ulcer, an occasional complication of cortisone therapy, and we had to discontinue the medicine. Finally, despite all we had done, Louise's knees became so stiff and sore that she needed crutches to get around and even used a wheelchair when she was home. She was becoming despondent.

Now, however, it was 1972 and the artificial knees— metallic prostheses that could be substituted for the roughened ends of the bones in the knee joint—had become increasingly effective and reliable. The first metallic knee prosthesis had been developed in 1969 but, as is customary with new devices, time had proven that they weren't as satisfactory as the orthopedists had hoped. But over a very few years, surgical technique and engineering modifications in the structure of the prosthesis had rapidly improved the prosthesis. Now, in most cases, they could be substituted for worn-out knee joints to greatly decrease the pain and improve the mobility of patients crippled with osteoarthritis. It was time, I decided, to refer Louise to an orthopedic surgeon.

I explained the possibilities to her. I warned her that if the prosthesis got infected the results would be bad, and that the operation was still too new to guarantee improvement. I also told her that it was possible—even probable—that the operation would help. It might even make her very much better.

"Dr. Nolen," she said, "even if you told me the chances were only one in a thousand that I'd be helped, I'd want to take that chance. I don't want to spend the rest of my life in a wheelchair and that's what's going to happen if something isn't done."

So I referred Louise to an orthopedic surgeon in Minneapolis, one who had had extensive experience in the insertion of knee prostheses. (Orthopedic surgeons are beginning to subspecialize to a great degree. Where they are organized into groups, it's not uncommon to find one or two members who do all the knee prosthesis cases, while another may operate on all the hip prosthesis patients referred to the group. This seems to me a wise policy, since it enables one or two people to rapidly gain extensive experience with an operation.) He, of course, told her all the same things that I had told her and even showed her a prosthesis and explained how it worked, a practice appreciated by patients and their referring doctors.

In March 1972 Louise had her right knee operated on. The result was so satisfactory that she could hardly wait to have the left knee done, as it was ten weeks later. Two months after her second operation, in late-July 1972, Louise came walking into my office, without crutches and with a minimal limp that would go undetected unless the observer were looking for it. She was smiling broadly, obviously pleased with the result.

"Dr. Nolen," she said as she sat down, "I can't tell you how pleased I am. I'm a new woman. I'll bet you didn't even know that when I was young, before I had to work regularly and before my knees started to bother me, I used to play golf. Well, yesterday, for the first time in twenty years, I went out and played with a friend. Only three holes—I didn't want to overdo—but you can't imagine how great it felt to be able to walk again without pain. I feel like a new woman."

"You look like a new woman, Louise. You know," I added, "I don't think I've ever seen you smile before."

"I guess that's because I haven't had much to smile about," she said, "though that isn't true and I should be ashamed of myself for saying it. There were a lot of people worse off than me even when my knees were at their worst. I guess I just used to let it get me down when I was in here.

"Anyway, I feel wonderful now—the best in years—and even if it doesn't last long I'll be grateful for whatever time it does last."

Louise is now sixty-five, and though I haven't asked about her golf lately, I still see her occasionally in a grocery or a drugstore and she always tells me how well she's doing. "My knees hardly bother me at all, Dr. Nolen," she said just recently. "I'm retired now and all I do is occasionally babysit my grandson, but I can walk around town and up and down stairs without any trouble. I'm so glad that operation came along when I needed it."

"So am I, Louise," I said. "I'd have hated to see you stuck in a wheelchair just because of your knees when all the rest of you works so well."

Stories like Louise's are getting more common every day. Ever since the first total hip replacement was performed—by Dr. Charnley in 1960—steady progress has been made in the art and science of joint replacement. There are many thousands of people walking around comfortably on artificial hips in 1980 who, twenty-five years ago, would have been crippled and confined to wheelchairs or limited to struggling around on crutches.

I have a friend, a lawyer I'll call Pat, who is still in very active practice at eighty-one. He had to have a portion of his large intestine removed in 1972 because of cancer. At operation the surgeon found the cancer was confined to the bowel and afterward the surgeon told Pat that, though he wouldn't promise anything, the chance that he was cured was, in his estimation, at least ninety percent.

Pat loved to fish, hunt and play golf. Unfortunately, along with his bowel cancer, he also had severe degenerative arthritis of his right hip. He had already had to give up golf and hunting and could only fish when he could do so from a boat while someone else rowed.

"I said, 'to hell with this,' " he later told me, and he went to an orthopedist and asked for a total hip replacement, an operation that I had mentioned would help him. The orthopedist was reluctant since only six months earlier Pat had had the bowel cancer operation, but Pat was adamant and, after conferring with the surgeon who had removed Pat's bowel, the orthopedist performed the total hip replacement.

That was in 1972 when Pat was seventy-three years old. Now, at eighty-one, besides carrying on his law practice he fishes, hunts, plays golf and—something he waited till he was seventy-five to do—travels extensively. He and his wife, Sal, have been all over the world in the last six years and they've had a great time everywhere they've been. It's wonderful to see Pat able to enjoy life as thoroughly as he does.

In the last twenty years the strides in orthopedic surgery have been awesome. Surgical innovation has played one leading role in the new developments but an equally important role has been played by the chemists and metallurgists who have developed glues and metal products that the body tolerates and which will bear the stress that continued use puts on the products. Metal "fatigue," which earlier resulted in breaks, is no longer a problem with the new alloys available for use. Total artificial hips can be expected to bear up under stress and strain as long as the patient lives.

Now artificial finger joints are becoming widely used to replace the "burned out" joints of arthritic hands. Shoulders, elbows and ankles can also be replaced, though success with these joints is not as great as it is with the hips and knees.

One of the questions that is often asked is, "Isn't it expensive to replace hips and knees?"

The short-sighted answer is "yes." Let's say that in 1980 a total hip replacement, if we include hospital charges and the physicians' fees, totals $10,000. To most of us that is a lot of money.

But the long-sighted answer is, "No, it's a bargain." Because by replacing the hip—or any other joint—you enable the person who has had the operation to continue an active, productive life. Pat, for example, even with his current reduced work load, is still earning $50,000 a year in 1980. He pays taxes, supports himself and his wife, and continues to be a valuable asset to our society. In the eight years since his operation his contribution to society has been about fifty times greater than the initial investment in his surgery.

Think of Louise. If she had to go on Social Security and welfare at the age of fifty-seven, which would have been the case had she not had her knee replacements, society would have had to bear the financial burden of support for her and at least some of her family for the last eight years. Instead of a burden, she has been, and continues to be, an asset to our society.

People who say society "can't afford" medical advances not only aren't thinking in terms of the cost in misery that the disease victim pays; they aren't even thinking in terms of financial value. I can't think of a single medical advance that has cost society anywhere near as much money as it has saved.

And if that weren't true, I'd still be all for the advances. Seeing the happiness that progress has brought to people like Louise and Pat makes me believe that the operations would be cheap at any price.

21

The Gift of Life

Lori Moran was born in 1955. She is the third child of Jean and Ray Moran. Their other two children are Mary, who is two years older than Lori, and Michael, who is five years older.

Jean Moran, who had worked part-time as a dental technician till her third child was born, was—like all parents—very grateful to have healthy children. Ray, a stockbroker, agreed. As a father fortunate enough to have six healthy children, I know how often Joan and I say to ourselves and to each other—particularly when we're concerned about college expenses, little difficulties our children get into (minor car accidents, marijuana, beer) and all the trials and tribulations that are part of raising a family—"Well, we can at least thank the Lord they're healthy." We all know families in which one or more children have crippling, irremediable defects, and just thinking of the problems these parents cope with every day makes us feel guilty when we start feeling sorry for ourselves.

Jean Moran is one of those conscientious mothers who keeps a close watch on her children's health. She has a little notebook in which she records the dates when various immunizations were given; which of the common childhood diseases, such as chicken pox, that each child has had; which one is allergic to what. (Frankly,

we don't have such a book. I think Joan started to keep
these records once but within a few weeks either the
notebook got lost or she just gave up on it. When Billy
left for medical school in the fall of 1979, we couldn't
find any record that he'd ever had a complete series of
polio immunizations, though both Joan and I seem to
remember that he did a few years ago when the school
program was going on. A doctor's children are often
like the proverbial shoeless children of the shoemaker;
they don't always get optimum medical care.)

The Moran children, who I knew casually because
they are about the same ages as three of my children,
were all healthy and thriving until 1960 when Lori, the
baby of the family who was then five, got a strep throat.
Jean didn't believe in bothering the doctor with every
little ailment her children had (nor would I), but when
Lori mentioned after five days that her throat still hurt,
Jean brought her in to see Dr. Jim Robinson (pseu-
donym), a local G.P. Jim took a look at her throat,
found it to be unusually red and sore-looking, so,
before starting Lori on penicillin, he took a throat
culture. (Often doctors don't bother with throat
cultures because of the added cost to the patient and
because, in most instances, the throat infection will have
cleared up on antibiotics by the time the report comes
back. If Lori's throat hadn't been quite so red and
swollen, Jim Robinson wouldn't have cultured it.)

The penicillin cleared Lori's throat up in three days.
But to make certain that the infection was completely
gone, Jim kept her on penicillin a full week. When the
culture report came back it showed streptococcus of the
A beta-hemolytic type. This is the strain of streptococcus that used to cause scarlet fever, a disease we
rarely see now that antibiotics are so widely used to treat
throat infections. Fortunately, the streptococcus, unlike
the staphylococcus, has never developed any significant
ability to resist penicillin.

Three weeks after Lori's attack of strep throat, she

woke up one morning and noticed that the skin of her fingers and around her eyes was puffy. She reported these things to her mother, though it was hardly necessary to do so since the puffiness was obvious, and her mother called Dr. Robinson. An analysis of Lori's urine showed red blood cells and albumin, a protein that filters from the blood through the kidneys when the patient's kidneys are not functioning properly. Dr. Robinson did a few more blood tests and had Lori examined by an internist who was a subspecialist on kidney diseases; their conclusion was that Lori had acute glomerulonephritis, an inflammation of the kidneys that sometimes develops anywhere from seven days to three weeks after an infection with A beta-hemolytic streptococci.

No one knows the exact cause of acute glomerulonephritis. Because of the length of time that elapses between the acute streptococcal infection and the kidney disease, it's believed that the latter may be a type of delayed allergic reaction to the streptococcus. Often the patient who develops acute glomerulonephritis won't even remember having had a previous streptococcal infection. Only after diligent questioning will the patient recall that a few weeks before he noticed the puffiness of his face or blood in his urine, he did have a minor "scratchy" throat for a few days. In these cases it can't be proven that the patient had a strep throat, but in all probability he did.

About ninety percent of children and at least sixty percent of adults who develop acute glomerulonephritis following strep infection will get well over a two- or three-week period. They may stay puffy for a short while, pass small amounts of blood in their urine and perhaps, transiently, develop high blood pressure, but as the acute reaction subsides their symptoms and their kidney function return to normal.

Unfortunately, some patients aren't so lucky. Instead of returning to normal their kidneys continue to deteriorate, and the patient acquires what is called chronic glomerulonephritis. As months go by, the kidney cells that usually excrete waste matter and excessive salt, and that keep the blood constituents at acceptable levels and maintain normal blood pressure, shrivel up, die and are replaced by scar tissue. By regulating diet, using medications and combating infections when and if they arise, the patient can usually live in reasonable comfort as long as at least a moderate amount of healthy kidney tissue remains; enough to eliminate the waste products that accumulate in the bloodstream as a natural result of normal metabolic processes. But unfortunately, as the years go by the natural course of chronic glomerulonephritis leads to a situation in which the kidneys can no longer function well enough to maintain the patient's life and well-being. Until the artificial kidney was developed in the early 1940's and kidney transplantation became feasible (in 1954), the end of the patient's kidney function meant the end of his life.

Lori, unfortunately, was one of the ten percent of children who went on to develop chronic glomerulonephritis. For the next twelve years, from 1960 till 1972, under the management of Dr. Robinson and the specialist in kidney diseases, Lori was able to live a near-normal life. She remained a bright, enthusiastic girl. She was an honor student and became a very good swimmer on the high school team. But in 1972 her kidney function had deteriorated so badly that she was barely excreting any urine at all. At that time, after discussing the situation with Lori and all of her family, agreement was reached that in order to continue to live—and to live a full life—Lori would either have to go on dialysis or have a kidney transplant. Dialysis is a process in which the patient's blood is filtered through an artificial kidney three times a week, usually for about six or eight hours each time. When the artificial kidney was first developed, problems with blood clotting, infection and rather rapid deterioration of the patient's health were common. By 1972, the cumbersome dialysis machines had been modified so that they were now more compact, less likely to cause infection, and relatively convenient for the patient to use. Many patients who originally had to go to hospitals to have their dialysis done were now able to use machines designed for home use with relatively little risk. In 1979 these compact machines have been improved even further and it is expected that most dialysis patients will be able to live many years, perhaps a near-normal life span, using the machine three evenings a week.

But now Lori was seventeen years old, ready to go away to college and, if she could have her choice, she preferred to have an artificial kidney implanted into her body so that she wouldn't be tied down to the three-time-a-week dialysis regimen. Her doctors agreed, as did her family, and so in 1972 Dr. Robinson referred Lori to the University of Minnesota Hospital where, under the direction of Dr. John Najarian, the Chairman of the Department of Surgery since 1967, there is a kidney transplant program that is, by the common consent of almost all surgical departments in the United States, one of the best in the world. (Dr. Najarian told me in an interview in August 1979 that his transplant division had done about 1300 kidney transplants since 1967 and that they expect to perform about 168 transplants in 1979, more than in any other surgical center in the United States.)

In June 1972 Lori, her parents, and her brother and sister were first seen by the transplant team, both medical and surgical specialists at the University. After reviewing Lori's history and reading over the records that had been forwarded to the University by Dr. Robinson, the transplant team agreed that, if a suitable donor could be found, Lori was an excellent candidate for a transplant. Despite her long history of progressive kidney failure she was in essentially excellent health. She was admitted to the hospital for a few days so that a very thorough examination could be done—including special blood tests which we'll get to later—and during these few days she was visited by a psychiatrist to make certain that she had the emotional stability to accept a transplant. This is a routine practice in most hospitals, particularly when the patient is under eighteen.

In the meantime, the transplant team interviewed Lori's parents, brother and sister to see if any of them would be willing to serve as a donor. All of them were willing and so tests were done on each to see which one, if any, was the closest "match." The success rate in kidney transplants is usually, though not invariably, related to how closely the donor's tissues resemble the recipient's. It is possible to transplant a kidney from one identical twin to another almost with impunity. Unless some surgical technical error is made—or a clot develops in the artery of the kidney when it is attached to the artery of the recipient—the transferred kidney should begin to function immediately and do so indefinitely, without the need to use the antirejection drugs that other transplant patients (those who do not have an identical twin donor) take all their lives.

For a person to serve as a donor several things are necessary.

First, the donor must be healthy.

Second, the donor must have the same blood type as the recipient, particularly as far as the major types are concerned. (We usually think of a patient as being a type A, B, O or AB; and Rh negative or positive. Actually there are many other subtypes within these groups, but usually they are not of major consequence.)

Third, the tissue type of the donor—the antigens (proteins) of the donor's cells—should match those of the recipient as closely as possible. Identical twins have identical tissue antigens. When the potential donor is not an identical twin, then four major antigens which are part of the lymphocytes (a species of blood cell) are typed and compared with those of the recipient. If all four antigens match, the chances of a successful transplant run near ninety percent; if three of the four antigens match, the chance for success drops to about seventy percent. If less than three antigens match, the donor is considered unacceptable, unless no better donor can be found.

The chances of a good match between siblings is higher than it is between parents and child. After all, the children got all their genes (and antigens) from both parents, while a child shares only half his genes with his mother, the other half with his father. (I don't want to make this too complicated, so I'll let the explanation rest there.)

It turned out that in Lori's case the match between her and her brother Michael was excellent; both had the same blood type and all four lymphocyte antigens matched. Michael was in excellent health and eager to donate a kidney to his sister.

Let me make it very clear that an individual requires only one kidney to live a full, active life. Assuming the operation on Michael was a success—as in any major operation, there is a risk of complications and even death (far less than one percent) when a kidney is removed—Michael would be able to live a completely active, normal life with one kidney. However, he would have to accept the fact that if his remaining kidney was either seriously damaged in an accident, or developed a disease (severe infection or a cancer) which required its removal, then he would have to go on dialysis or have a transplant himself.

The decision to become a donor is not one to be made lightly and at the University of Minnesota every effort is made to explain all the possible consequences, however remote, of kidney donation. Under no circumstances is pressure even brought to bear on anyone to make him or her feel guilty if he or she chooses not to be a donor. (I discussed this subject at great length with Ms. Justine Willmert, a nurse who agreed to move from San Francisco to the University of Minnesota when Dr. Najarian became Chairman in 1967 because, as Dr. Najarian told me, "Justine knows more about transplants than most doctors. I didn't see how I could have gotten this program really going without her help." Among the many things she told me was that when a transplanted kidney fails to function, as sometimes happens even with the best matches, the donor often feels guilty. "He or she blames her or himself for the failure," Justine told me. "The problem is particularly severe when the donor was a reluctant donor; those donors really get down on themselves. They feel that because they weren't really anxious to help their brother or sister or parent—maybe just out of fear—that they and their relative are being punished. I try to screen out all reluctant donors. There's no disgrace in being afraid to go through a major operation on behalf of someone else."

Michael was not a reluctant donor. Even after Justine had explained all the possibilities to him, he was willing, even eager, to donate a kidney to Lori. The Morans had always been a very close family and they were never closer than they were in June of 1972.

In 1980 a patient who needs a transplant, even if there is an acceptable donor available, has to wait about three months to have the operation performed at the University of Minnesota Hospital. Kidney donors and recipients require very close preoperative, operative and postoperative care so, in 1980, Dr. Najarian finds it impractical and potentially unsafe to do more than three elective transplants a week. The total number of transplants done is greater than this, because there is a list of about 200 patients who have no suitable donor, and when a donor does become available—perhaps as the result of a car accident which produced a brain dead patient whose family is willing to allow the University team to remove and transplant their relative's healthy organs—the patient on the waiting list who best matches the donor is called immediately to the hospital and the

operation is done as an emergency. Once kidneys are
removed from a donor they are suitable for transplantation for only seventy-two hours, even if the kidneys are constantly perfused with a nutrient solution.
(The perfusion pump was developed at the University of
Minnesota and either the original pump, or a model
based on the original design, are now used world-wide,
wherever kidney transplants are done.) When a donor
kidney becomes available, if it can't be used in the
hospital where the patient died, perhaps because the
hospital does not have a transplant service, the kidney is
immediately shipped to a hospital where there is a
recipient on the waiting list whose tissues closely match
those of the donor.

Ordinarily an acceptable match can be found at a
relatively nearby hospital. However, once in a while the
antigens of the donor will be so unusual that there is no
suitable recipient in the area. In that case the information (blood and tissue type) is fed into a computer. Rarely will there be no one in the entire country
who is a suitable recipient for this kidney. In that case
an international search is carried out. (There is a computer at The Hague in the Netherlands into which the
names and blood and tissue types of all potential
recipients have been programmed.) Dr. Najarian told
me that on one occasion they were offered the kidney
from a brain-dead patient in Finland. "His antigens
didn't match any waiting recipient in England or
Europe," he said, "but they were a near-perfect match
for a farmer from North Dakota. So while a doctor
from Finland flew to Minnesota with the kidney, we
flew in the farmer from North Dakota and had him
ready for operation when the kidney arrived. The doctor from Finland got held up in some sort of mix-up at
Kennedy Airport, but we still managed to get the kidney
transplanted within seventy-two hours.

"Incidentally," Dr. Najarian continued, "the North
Dakota farmer was Finnish too. We find that situation

often. People of the same race are apt to make the best matches. Around here with all the Scandinavians, it's best to be a Swede or a Norwegian if you need a graft."

In 1972 the waiting list of patients with suitable donors was very short and, once the preliminary work-up had been completed, Dr. Najarian scheduled Lori's transplant operation to be done two weeks later.

Early on the morning of July 17, 1972, Lori Moran was sedated and wheeled into one of the special operating rooms reserved for transplant patients at the University. Her brother, Michael, was wheeled into a nearby operating room. After both patients had been anesthetized, one operating team operated on Michael, exposing his left kidney with a long segment of the artery which supplied the kidney with blood, an equally long segment of the vein which drained the kidney and several inches of the ureter (the tube through which urine flows from the kidney to the bladder). When I write a "long segment" of the kidney artery and vein, the term is relative. Those blood vessels are only about two inches long, so the surgeon removes the artery right from the point where it originates from the aorta.

At the same time, a second team of surgeons began to operate on Lori. Customarily, if a left kidney is removed from the donor it is implanted into the pelvis on the right side of the recipient, so it was the right pelvic area, down in Lori's groin, which was exposed. The big vessels that run from the abdomen down to the leg were exposed as well as Lori's urinary bladder. As soon as Lori's pelvis was adequately exposed, the surgical team operating on Michael removed the kidney with its artery, vein and ureter and they were immediately placed in a sterile metal basin and brought into the room where the surgeons were operating on Lori. Since both surgical teams had performed these operations many times before, it took them only about ten minutes to attach the artery and vein of Michael's kidney to a large artery and vein (the internal iliac artery and the iliac vein) in Lori. Within three minutes after Michael's kidney was attached to Lori's blood vessels the donated kidney began producing urine. The ureter of Michael's kidney was then implanted in Lori's bladder and the wound was closed.

While the kidney implantation was being done the surgical team assigned to Michael had already closed his wound and he had been transferred to the recovery room. About half an hour later Lori was in the room reserved for patients who had just had transplants. She would be monitored very closely, by both nurses and doctors, for the next few days to make certain not only that her new kidney continued to function but that her general health remained normal. There would be a critical period a few hours or days after the operation in which her body might attempt to reject Michael's kidney—a so-called hyperacute rejection—and for the rest of her life she would have to take medicines (immuran and cortisone) which would make less likely the chance that her body would "recognize" Michael's kidney as "foreign" and reject it, but with careful monitoring these risks were not great. At the very worst—if rejection began and could not be stopped by increased drug dosages and/or X-ray—she would lose the kidney and require dialysis. With such a good tissue match the hope was that none of these things would happen.

They haven't. At least not as of 1980. Michael was out of the hospital a week after he had donated his kidney; Lori remained three weeks longer because, as recently as 1972, transplant surgeons worried more about their patients than they do now that they have more experience.

Lori is now twenty-four years old. She graduated from college two years ago and teaches in a school not far from Litchfield. She takes four pills a day, returns to the University of Minnesota once a year for a general checkup, but otherwise leads a normal life. Her first child was born six months ago and is completely healthy. Michael, who is twenty-seven, is a consulting engineer with a firm in Chicago. He too is married and is the father of three young children. All things considered, an extremely happy ending to what would have been a fatal disease twenty years ago.

But is it the ending? I asked this question of John Najarian in August 1979. "We certainly hope it is," he said. "We've now got several transplant patients who have lived comfortable, productive lives for over seventeen years—as you can see, I'm including some we operated on back in California before I came here—but even in the twelve years I've been in Minnesota, I can think offhand of a dozen or more who have lived over ten years. With the things we've learned even in the last couple of years, we expect we'll have many very long-term survivals; I'd use the word 'cures' but until we unravel the entire secret of rejection I guess that would be premature."

"Weren't you worried about your transplant patients getting pregnant?" I asked. "I'd think that with the drugs they take you'd be worried about deformed fetuses, to say nothing of the kidney problems that even normal pregnant women have."

"Sure, we were worried," Dr. Najarian said, "but how do you stop people from getting pregnant? You can't pass a law forbidding it.

"Anyway, to our great delight the women with transplanted kidneys who have had babies have done very nicely. Over a hundred have had post-transplant babies and as far as we can tell, the incidence of even minor deformities in the infant is no higher than in the normal population.

"We also worried that the immuran (a drug that suppresses rejection) might make our male recipients sterile, but that hasn't happened either. A number of them have become fathers. We're all very pleased.

"Right now our results are pretty darn good—five-year transplanted kidney survival is running about eighty percent—and I haven't any doubt that figure will improve substantially. We've learned some new tricks, simply by experience. For one thing, we recently discovered that patients who had had several transfusions before transplantation did better than those who hadn't had any, probably because their bodies had developed a greater tolerance for foreign cells. Now we give five transfusions—one quarter of a pint of blood from five different donors—to each recipient a few weeks before operation. I think that is going to help.

"And I'm very excited about a new technique we've developed for transplanting part of the pancreas. Right now we only do this in severe diabetics who have already had a kidney transplant, but we've got one patient who was completely dependent on insulin shots before surgery and hasn't needed one injection since her transplant, which we did more than a year ago.

"You know that the five-year survival with heart transplants is up over fifty percent now and that Tom Starzl down in Denver is getting better results all the time with his liver transplantations. I'm very optimistic that with all the research going on—you know we've got at least a half dozen labs here working on various phases of the transplant problem—we'll be saving thousands of patients a year with transplants in the very near future. It's a fascinating field."

John Najarian and Justine Willmert are both outspoken people but they're also realists. They've been working in the field of transplantation a long time. If they think it's a promising field, I'm inclined to agree.

Lori Moran's case is just one of the many that have helped convince me.

22

Let's Hear It for
the House Call!

On a Friday evening in September 1975 Joan and I came home at 11:00 P.M., after having gone out to dinner. I had just put on my pajamas, mixed myself a nightcap and was sitting down to read the evening newspaper, when our phone rang. "Damn it," I said, "can't I have any peace?" Joan didn't bother to answer my question, having heard me ask it at least twenty thousand times over the last twenty-six years. I got up and answered the phone.

(I might note here that one of the best investments I have ever made was one I made in 1966 when the oldest of our children was twelve. Our children had begun to receive many phone calls about that time and, since I always curse either silently or out loud, depending on the company and my mood, whenever the phone rings, I decided then to put in a second set of telephones with a different sounding ring—chimes—for the children. Their extensions are in the basement and in what is laughingly referred to as "Dad's study." Our phone extensions—Joan's and mine—are in the dining room and in our bedroom. In the local phone directory there is a listing for "Nolen kids." Their phone could ring till the house shook and it wouldn't upset me a bit. But when

my phone rings I'm sure a little extra acid pours out of
my stomach cells, my blood pressure probably goes up
twenty points and, at the very least, I utter "damn."
The stress that second set of telephones saves me
should, if all the theories regarding stress are correct,
add years to my life.)

On this particular night the call was from a woman
I'll call Frieda Morgan. She and her husband, Jim, who
was fifty-eight at the time, have been good friends of
ours ever since we moved to Litchfield. We often see
them socially and Jim and I often play tennis together.

"Bill," Frieda said, "I hope I didn't wake you up. I
know you don't like to make house calls, but I wonder if
you'd make an exception this time. Jim has been in bed
all afternoon with a sore belly and he refuses to see
anyone but you. I knew you and Joan were going to
Minneapolis this afternoon and out to dinner tonight
and I wanted him to go to the clinic and see someone
else, but you know how stubborn he is. I just couldn't
convince him. I've been calling off and on all day. I hate
to ask you to come out at this late hour, but I'm
worried. It's not like Jim to spend an afternoon in
bed."

To say that I don't like to make house calls is about as
great an understatement as anyone could make. In that
respect I am a perfectly typical doctor. I prefer to
examine patients in my office or at the hospital where
professional assistance and special diagnostic equipment is available if I should need it. But, and I feel very
strongly about this, I believe that there are times when a
doctor ought to make house calls—for example, in a
situation where a child wakes up at two in the morning
crying because of an earache which the doctor can
probably diagnose and treat with ease at the patient's
home—and on occasions such as this one, where the
patient is so stubborn that if the doctor doesn't go to
him, he won't receive any medical care.

I assured Frieda that she hadn't wakened me. I didn't

tell her that I was in my pajamas about to relax with a drink. Instead I simply said, "Tell your stubborn ox of a husband I'll be there in ten minutes."

When I got there Jim was lying on his bed and didn't appear, at first glance, to be very sick. "What's the problem, Jim?" I asked.

"I don't really know, Bill," he said. "It's just that my stomach is sore. It's been bothering me off and on for a couple of months. Mostly just a dull ache, low, down here," and he pointed to a spot just below his navel. "Sometimes it's worse than others, but there's nothing special I notice that makes it worse. Sometimes it almost feels like it's throbbing, almost like I had my heart in my belly. I had some blood in my bowel movement about a month ago and I thought maybe I was just constipated. I tried taking a laxative but it didn't help.

"Then this noon it got really sore. It even began to bother me in the back so I could hardly walk. That's when I decided to go to bed.

"I've tried both a heating pad and an ice bag on it, but neither one helped. I've had about six aspirin and two Valiums that Frieda had left from that time she was having nerve problems. They cut down on the pain some, but I think I need something stronger."

"Slow down, Jim," I said. "Before I give you anything stronger I want to figure out what you've got. Let me feel that belly of yours." I put my hand on the upper part of his abdomen and pushed gently.

"It's not up there, Bill," Jim said, "it's down here." Again, he pointed to an area below his navel.

"I know that, Jim," I said, "it's just that I want to press first where it doesn't hurt. We'll get to the sore area later." This is the routine most doctors use in examining an abdomen. Start where it doesn't hurt, just so the patient can get used to your examining hand and you can get a sense of what his normal abdominal wall feels like; then move to the tender area.

Which is what I did a few seconds later and, almost immediately, I was sure of the diagnosis. Jim was slightly obese, weighing about 210 pounds at a height of six feet, so there was probably about an inch of fat beneath his skin and another inch of abdominal muscle. Still, beneath these, I could feel a pulsating lump which I estimated was about the size of an apple. When I pressed on it gently, Jim winced. I took my stethoscope out of my pocket and placed it on Jim's abdomen, over the lump. Through it I could hear a "whooshing" sound like that which water makes as it flows through a rusty pipe. I was virtually certain that Jim had what is known as an aneurysm of the aorta.

The aorta is the largest blood vessel in the body. It begins at the heart, curves around in the upper chest, and then runs down the front of the spine to a point just below the navel where it bifurcates (i.e., divides) into two main trunks called the common iliacs. These trunks divide again. One branch flows into the pelvis and the other runs down the thigh and supplies blood, after further subdividing, to the leg.

As the aorta runs from the heart down along the spine through the chest and abdomen, many arteries, some small, some relatively large, spread out from it like branches from a tree trunk. For example, two large arteries—the carotid arteries—arise from the aorta shortly after it leaves the heart. The arteries to the kidneys arise from the aorta about two inches above the point where it bifurcates into the two common iliacs and it is in this area that the aorta is most likely to balloon out into what we call an aneurysm. The aneurysm wall is lined by arteriosclerotic plaques and as the aorta pulsates, as it does with each beat of the heart, the aneurysm will, sometimes in months, sometimes not for years, gradually dilate as the wall begins to thin and weaken from recurrent internal pressure. Sometimes the aorta, which is normally about one and a half inches in diameter at this point, will expand till its diameter is six or seven inches. Often, however, before it reaches such an enormous size it will simply explode, blood will spurt out through the hole in the aneurysm, and unless the patient is operated on immediately he will almost certainly die of this internal hemorrhage.

As I went over Jim's story with him once more, it seemed almost certain that an aneurysm, which was either already leaking or was ready to explode, was the cause of his trouble. He had admitted that he had been at least occasionally aware of an abnormal pulsating mass in his abdomen for several months. The blood in his stool a few weeks earlier might have come from a small leak from the aneurysm into the adjacent bowel, and his relatively new back pain probably meant that the aneurysm was now beginning to erode the vertebrae of the lower spine. All this was speculation, of course, but the history and the physical examination fit the picture of an abdominal aortic aneurysm so well that I had no doubt my diagnosis was correct.

The only question was how to treat him; the aneurysm might blow out in an hour, or twelve hours, or even a week. But the probability that it would blow and do so relatively soon seemed to me highly likely. I thought Jim ought to have his aneurysm operated on very soon.

I have operated on only two aneurysms in the twenty years I've been in practice. Both were operations performed after the aneurysms had blown open. One patient lasted three days; one died on the operating room table. Fifteen years ago, when I had done my most recent abdominal aneurysm operation, the mortality in patients whose aneurysms had blown prior to surgery was almost ninety percent. Now, in the hands of experienced vascular surgeons, the mortality is lower but still not much better than forty percent. I still fish blood clots out of arteries when necessary—a relatively small operation that has to be done as an emergency to save a limb—but I stay away from the fancy stuff.

So the answer to the question, "Should I operate on Jim?" was, in my opinion, a very emphatic "No." That decision reached, I explained to Frieda and Jim what the diagnosis was and what I proposed to do.

I explained to them what an aneurysm was. I told them that ordinarily the operation could be carried out, with a very low mortality rate, perhaps one or two percent, provided the patient's aneurysm hadn't blown open and that the patient was in otherwise good health; both conditions existed in Jim's case. I explained, drawing sketches as I did so, how in the ordinary operation for abdominal aneurysms the surgeon puts clamps across the aorta above and below the aneurysm, cuts out the aneurysm, and replaces this section of worn out aorta with a hollow tube made of Teflon or some other synthetic material. Sometimes a straight piece of tubing is all that is necessary. However, if the aneurysm extends into the first portion of the common iliacs, then the surgeon would use an inverted Y-shaped piece of tubing sewing the upper, wider limb to the aorta and the lower two limbs to the iliacs. Technically, it usually isn't a difficult operation, unless the aorta has blown open or the aorta or iliacs above and below the aneurysm are in very poor condition due to arteriosclerosis. In some centers—particularly in Houston, where Dr. Michael DeBakey works—thousands of such operations are done each year; but in almost every major city there are now dozens of surgeons who "specialize" in vascular surgery.

"Can't you do the operation here in Litchfield?" Jim asked.

"I could do it," I said. "I always have a few pieces of Teflon tubing around in case I have to do the operation. But, to be truthful, my mortality rate as of 1975 is a hundred percent. You might be my first success but, as long as my hand isn't forced—as long as you're not in shock and not obviously hemorrhaging—I have no desire to try for my first local success.

"Nor do I want to send you to someone who does occasional aneurysms, with occasional successes; there are a few of these surgeons around. I think it's well worth the extra time to send you to Minneapolis to a surgeon I know who specializes in this sort of work and to whom we've sent other patients on whom he has operated successfully. It's up to you, of course, but frankly, Jim, I don't think you have any reasonable alternative. I think we'd better send you to Minneapolis."

"When would I go? In the morning?"

"In the morning, yes, if you consider 12:15 A.M. morning. That's about how long it will take the ambulance to get here after I've called my surgical friend and made arrangements for your transfer."

"You think it's that urgent?" Frieda asked.

"If I didn't, Frieda," I said, "I wouldn't wake my surgeon friend up at midnight to tell him about Jim. I suspect he'll have Jim on the operating table within a couple of hours of the time Jim's in Minneapolis."

"Darn," Jim said, "and to think I expected all I'd need was an enema."

We all had a chuckle. It broke the tension.

So I called my friend John in Minneapolis, told him of Jim's symptoms and my physicial examination, and he said, "Send him right down. It sounds as if that thing might blow any time. I'll meet him at the hospital. How long do you figure it will be?"

"A couple of hours," I said, "and let me know what you find." I arranged for the ambulance to come, wished Jim well, and got to bed about 1:00 A.M.

The next morning at 11:00 A.M. John called me. "I just finished operating, Bill," he said. "It's amazing your friend Jim even survived to call you. That aneurysm measured six inches in diameter. A big part of the back wall was gone but, luckily, there was so much scar tissue that the side walls were stuck to the vertebrae. I had to put in a Y graft, since it involved the upper ends of both iliacs.

"He tolerated the operation beautifully, at least so far. I don't anticipate any trouble. I was able to stay below the renal arteries [aneurysms rarely extend above the renal arteries, the arteries to the kidneys] and he's making urine already. If everything goes well he ought to be out of here in a week."

"Great, John," I said. "He's a close friend and a hell of a nice guy. I'm glad you could help him."

"Next time," John said, "why don't you send me someone in the afternoon? I like to go at these things leisurely."

"Next time," I said, "maybe I won't make the house call. Then you won't have to get out of bed at all."

Jim was home in a week. He had lost a few pounds, which he could spare, and he was on some pills for his high blood pressure—a factor that had probably contributed to the development of his aneurysm—but within two months he was back at his law practice, full time. He hasn't had any trouble in the five years since his operation.

There are, I suppose, two lessons that could be learned from Jim's case. The first, and most impressive to a surgeon who started training in 1953, is how far we've advanced in the field of vascular surgery since the first abdominal aortic graft was done by Du Bost of Paris in 1940.

At Bellevue, in 1953 and even in 1957, we would often argue at surgical conferences whether it was better to leave a large aortic aneurysm in a patient alone or operate and remove it. In those days we used mostly aortic grafts taken from cadavers, though the synthetic grafts were just coming into use. The mortality rate was so high, even in the most capable hands, that there was a real question whether there would be a net gain or loss in years of survival if we operated on aneurysms discovered during routine physical examinations, even including those aneurysms that were causing symptoms.

Now, unless the patient is so very old or so enfeebled

by other diseases that he or she couldn't possibly tolerate the surgery, there is no question that any doctor would recommend removal of an abdominal aneurysm. The mortality ought to be less than five percent in elective cases, and once the operation has been done, the patient's life expectancy is essentially what it would be in someone without an artificial aorta.

Moreover, we are now using synthetic grafts (or vein grafts) to improve the blood supply to vessels in the legs, the abdomen, even the brain. Vascular surgeons routinely perform these operations with marked improvement in the patient's well-being. Vascular surgery, though it is not formally recognized as such, is in fact a specialty to which many surgeons devote most of their time. (Beware, as I said earlier, of the general surgeon who does an "occasional" vascular case. Vascular surgeons may have to do occasional general surgical cases, since there aren't enough candidates for blood vessel surgery to keep all trained, would-be vascular surgeons busy, but the reverse does not apply.)

The second, and possibly more widely applicable point, is this. The doctor who always refuses to make house calls, who tells patients who call him after 9:00 P.M. to "take two aspirin and see me in the morning," is, eventually, going to be responsible for someone's death.

As I can't say too emphatically: I hate house calls but I make them. Not at every request—often all the caller needs is the reassurance that I feel safe in giving over the phone—but whenever I'm in doubt I either make the house call or have the patient meet me at the hospital, whichever seems most appropriate.

I've tried the "take two aspirin and see me in the morning" routine, and for me (to say nothing of the patient) it doesn't work. I turn over and try to get back to sleep while wondering if what I think is most likely indigestion might not be a heart attack. Or I think about that cold foot that old Mr. Smith suddenly noticed and it occurs to me that maybe it isn't just his old age and poor circulation; maybe he has thrown a clot from his heart to a leg artery and maybe by the time I see him in the morning his leg will be beyond salvage and require amputation; so, after tossing for five or ten minutes, I invariably call the patient back, get dressed and go on the house call. I only thank the Lord that in 1980 not many patients ask me to make house calls. In Meeker County it's known that I'm a surgeon and it's the G.P.s who get the house call requests.

For Jim's sake—and my own—this was one call I'm glad I made.

Epilogue

Progress in medicine is sometimes slow, sometimes amazingly fast. Usually, however, if you look carefully at the so-called "breakthroughs" in medicine, the events that produce headlines, you find that they came as the end result of a great deal of tedious, painstaking work, much of it done by technicians who never share in the glory of the person or persons who finally announce the "breakthrough."

Consider, for example, the first successful heart transplant performed by Christiaan Barnard in 1967. His achievement was based on work that went back at the very least to 1907, when Alexis Carrel, a French scientist who by then had emigrated to the United States, developed a technique for suturing blood vessels together, enabling surgeons to perform the first animal to animal transplants. Carrel was, in fact, honored; he received the Nobel Prize in 1912.

To dwell for a few more moments on the transplant for which Barnard received so much adulation. His accomplishment wouldn't have been possible unless Dr. John Gibbon of Jefferson Medical School in Pennsylvania had spent years working in a laboratory trying to develop the heart-lung machine which made it possible to sustain life while the heart was stopped. Dozens of other surgeons, and innumerable unsung technicians, also spent years working toward this goal. Dr. Barnard got ninety-nine percent of the credit for his achievement (and he certainly deserved a share of the plaudits), but his actual contribution to all that was necessary to this ultimate achievement was certainly only a fraction of one percent. (I suspect that Dr. Barnard would agree with this statement.)

Often achievements in medicine are the results of chance. The story of Alexander Fleming and his discovery of penicillin—the first of the antibiotics which have revolutionized medical care, making infectious diseases far less lethal than they so recently were—has been recounted so often that it has become a part of medical folklore. Briefly, Fleming noticed that a bit of mold had accidentally fallen onto an agar plate in which he was culturing bacteria, and around the mold was a clear area. The mold was penicillium and it was destroying the bacteria. This observation led Fleming logically and quickly to the conclusion that penicillium might cure at least some patients afflicted with infectious diseases. This proved to be the case.

Fleming might have ignored the contaminating mold and its effect, in which case the development of antibiotics would probably have been significantly delayed. But Fleming was a scientist, a disciplined observer, and, to use a cliché, "chance favors the prepared mind."

The explosion in medical advances in the last fifty years has been truly amazing, but readily understandable. Scientific progress occurs in a geometric rather than arithmetic progression. As the base, the quantity of fundamental knowledge, widens, the chances of building higher on that base increase enormously. Science is not like art. In art individuals occasionally provide a base on which other individuals may build, but art is so personal, so unique, that the parallel between it and science is not very marked. Certainly, most playwrights can learn something about their field by reading Shakespeare, but to construct a better play than Shakespeare simply by adding to what he did is not realistic. The artist essentially works alone, and though he may in some vague way owe a debt to his predecessors, his accomplishments cannot be built upon theirs. In science—and medicine is both a science and an art—this can and is done.

As I write, in March 1980, medical/surgical help which we never dreamed would be available thirty years ago is now being offered in most of the major hospitals, and in many of the smaller hospitals, all across the United States. The coronary bypass operation, which restores blood flow to the heart by using veins or arteries to create detours around blocked arteries, was first performed in 1968. In 1980 it is estimated that at least 80,000 of these operations will be performed, restoring to active, pain-free, productive life patients who would once have been designated "coronary cripples" and be doomed to short, sedentary existences.

Advances in radiology have been so rapid that in 1975 the decision was made to divide the specialty into four separate areas. Now, following graduation from medical school, after three or four years of training you can become a specialist in diagnostic radiology, therapeutic radiology, nuclear radiology or special study radiology. Knowledge in these fields has grown so rapidly, that it is no longer possible to master all of what used to be called simply "radiology" in less than twelve years.

Orthopedics is growing with almost equal rapidity. It is not unusual in 1980 to find an orthopedic specialist who, as a recent announcement that came to my office said, "Specializes only in disorders of the leg, below the knee." Other orthopedists operate on nothing but hips; still others limit their practices only to the back. I will be very surprised if in a few years this current trend in orthopedics does not become a formal break into subspecialization.

At the same time, recognizing that someone must take care of the patient as a whole, lest we lose sight of personality and see only isolated organ problems, a relatively new subspecialty known as "Family Practice" has come into existence. The new medical graduates who want to practice continuing medical care, i.e., to take care of the same patients over many years, and to learn to manage perhaps eighty percent of all the ailments that plague the ordinary person in his sojourn through life. They also learn to recognize—and this is perhaps the most difficult job the family practitioner has—those diseases or disorders which should be referred to the doctors who specialize in only one segment of medical care. Family Practice, because it allows such a broad scope and fosters such close doctor-patient relationships, is a specialty which each year is attracting more and more young medical graduates.

Technology—the development of new metallic alloys, new synthetic sutures, new anticancer drugs, stronger and more bacterial-specific antibiotics—all these things have made recent practical advances in medicine possible. And as work continues in the research laboratories not only of hospitals but of pharmaceutical companies, electronic device manufacturers and computer companies, it is as certain as it can be that the medical revolution will continue, and in the not too distant future, diseases like cancer, multiple sclerosis, and arteriosclerosis will become as obsolete as smallpox, poliomyelitis and tuberculosis, which only a few years ago were the cause of so many deaths. Give up hope? Anyone whose memory goes back even ten years knows how foolish that would be.

As I hope these case studies have demonstrated, the greatest source of strength in medicine is the patient's own body. It is literally impossible to compare it, realistically, to a machine. The miraculous (and I choose the word intentionally) tasks that the liver, the brain, the kidney, the heart, the lungs—virtually every part of a human—perform every day can't be duplicated by even the most sophisticated computers. I suspect that in the overall design of the universe we are not intended to comprehend the limits of the human body. To do so would limit our ability to hope, in the face of what seems unavoidable disaster, for earthly salvation.

That hope, I have come to think, is perhaps the greatest of all God's gifts to us.

Bestsellers from Berkley
The books you've been hearing
about—and want to read

___**THE BEVERLY HILLS DIET**   05299-0—$3.50
    Judy Mazel
___**DADDY'S GIRL**   05172-2—$2.95
    Charlotte Vale Allen
___**DESTINIES**   05325-3—$3.25
    Charlotte Vale Allen
___**FAT IS A FEMINIST ISSUE**   05544-2—$2.95
    Susie Orbach
___**THE FIRST DEADLY SIN**   05604-X—$3.50
    Lawrence Sanders
___**MOMMIE DEAREST**   05242-7—$3.25
    Christina Crawford
___**PROMISES**   05502-7—$3.25
    Charlotte Vale Allen
___**SHADOWLAND**   05056-4—$3.50
    Peter Straub
___**THE TENTH COMMANDMENT**   05001-7—$3.50
    Lawrence Sanders
___**WARPATH** (Northwest Territory #1)   05452-1—$2.95
    Oliver Payne

Available at your local bookstore or return this form to:

 Berkley Book Mailing Service
P.O. Box 690
Rockville Centre, NY 11570

Please send me the above titles. I am enclosing $_____
(Please add 50¢ per copy to cover postage and handling). Send check or money
order—no cash or C.O.D.'s. Allow six weeks for delivery.

NAME_____

ADDRESS_____

CITY_____STATE/ZIP_____ 1J

More Bestsellers from Berkley
The books you've been hearing about and want to read

____ **CHILDREN OF DUNE**   05472-1—$2.75
Frank Herbert
____ **DUNE**   05471-3—$2.95
Frank Herbert
____ **DUNE MESSIAH**   05503-5—$2.75
Frank Herbert
____ **THE NEW ROGET'S THESAURUS
IN DICTIONARY FORM**   05723-2—$2.25
ed. by Norman Lewis
____ **THE SEARING**   04924-8—$2.95
John Coyne
____ **THE SECOND DEADLY SIN**   05545-0—$3.50
Lawrence Sanders
____ **THE SIXTH COMMANDMENT**   05504-3—$3.50
Lawrence Sanders
____ **WE ARE THE EARTHQUAKE
GENERATION**   04991-4—$2.75
Jeffrey Goodman
____ **WHISPERS**   04707-5—$2.95
Dean R. Koontz

Helpful... Candid...
Fascinating... Important...
Shocking... Timely...

...And Bestselling!

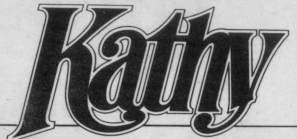